DIAGNOSTIC PICTURE TESTS IN

CARDIOLOGY

D.L.H. Patterson
MD, FRCP
Consultant Physician and Cardiologist
Islington and Bloomsbury Health Authorities
Whittington Hospital
London

Wolfe Medical Publications Ltd

Titles in this series, published or being developed, include:
Diagnostic Picture Tests in Paediatrics
Picture Tests in Human Anatomy
Diagnostic Picture Tests in Oral Medicine
Diagnostic Picture Tests in Orthopaedics
Diagnostic Picture Tests in Infectious Diseases
Diagnostic Picture Tests in Dermatology
Diagnostic Picture Tests in Ophthalmology
Diagnostic Picture Tests in Rheumatology
Diagnostic Picture Tests in Obstetrics/Gynaecology
Diagnostic Picture Tests in Clinical Neurology
Diagnostic Picture Tests in Injury in Sport
Diagnostic Picture Tests in General Surgery
Diagnostic Picture Tests in General Medicine
Diagnostic Picture Tests in Paediatric Dentistry
Diagnostic Picture Tests in Dentistry
Picture Tests in Embryology

Copyright © D.L.H. Patterson, 1989
First published in 1989 by Wolfe Medical Publications Ltd
Printed by W.S. Cowell Ltd, Ipswich, England
ISBN 0 7234 1622 2

For a full list of Wolfe Medical Atlases, plus
forthcoming titles and details of our surgical,
dental and veterinary Atlases, please write to
Wolfe Publishing Ltd, 2-16 Torrington Place,
London WC1E 7LT.

A CIP catalogue record for this book
is available from the British Library.

Preface

Most of these diagnostic picture tests are from patients presenting to a district general hospital. Some of the problems presented are common, other less so. The questions are intended to test knowledge at different levels of complexity; some invite a succinct answer, others are intended to produce a more discursive response. I hope this variety of questions and anticipated responses will serve to maintain the interest and stimulate the thought processes of the reader.

The techniques of non-invasive cardiology continue to increase the potential to refine the clinical assessment of a patient presenting with a cardiac problem. The cardiologist occupies a privileged position since any patient undergoing investigations will have them performed within the cardiac department under a watchful eye. A knowledge of such patients passing through the department is valuable from a number of points of view; not only does it enable the dissemination of information about the patient and the ability, if appropriate, to influence the subsequent management, but it is also a rich source of teaching material. I am grateful to the clinicians who requested these investigations. I am grateful also to the technicians and cardiographers who perform such a valuable function; their increasingly important role is unfortunately often not fully recognised.

Acknowledgements

I am grateful to all my colleagues for the referral of their patients for an investigation or for an opinion. I thank the following for providing illustrations: Professor P. Ell, Dr D. Grant, Dr J. Dyson, Dr A. Rubin and Dr G. Rubin.

For Gillian

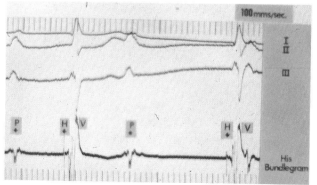

1 A surgeon has just taken the patient off bypass.
(a) What operation has been performed?
(b) What is the surgical mortality risk in a middle-aged man with stable symptoms?
(c) What is the duration of symptomatic benefit?

2 The recordings of the standard leads I, II, III together with the recording of the His bundle were obtained from a 36-year-old man who presents with tiredness.
(a) What is the rhythm?
(b) What do the H and V deflections represent?
(c) Is there any value in measuring the H-V interval and in what circumstances?

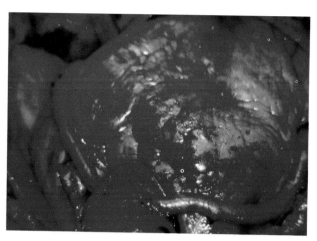

3

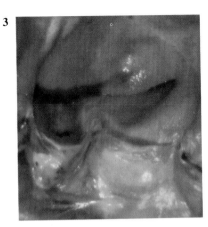

3 A picture of the aorta just above the aortic valve. The patient presented with chest pain and developed ventricular fibrillation in the Accident and Emergency department and could not be resuscitated.

(a) What is the likely cause of death?

(b) Why did the patient develop ventricular fibrillation?

(c) Are there any predisposing factors to this condition?

4 These pressures were recorded simultaneously with the ECG. The pulmonary artery wedge pressure and the left ventricular pressures are measured in mmHg; the scale is shown.

(a) What are the two main abnormalities and how severe is the condition?

(b) Name two serious complications of this condition.

(c) What might the pulmonary artery pressure be?

4

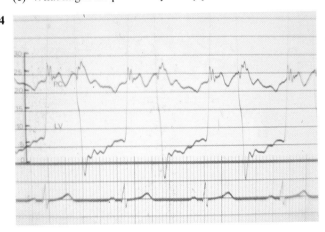

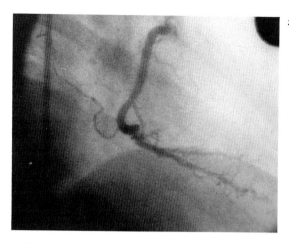

5 This view of a coronary arteriogram is taken in the right anterior oblique projection.
(a) Which coronary artery is it?
(b) Where does it run in the first part of its course?
(c) Name five of its main branches.

6 A 60-year-old woman complaining of progressively worsening shortness of breath had a heart murmur since the age of 24 years, when she was pregnant. She was not anaemic, was not in heart failure but had a tinge of cyanosis.
(a) Name four abnormalities in this x-ray.
(b) What lesion might account for them?
(c) What options are available to treat her symptoms?

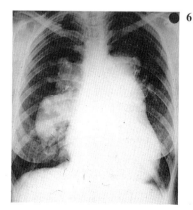

7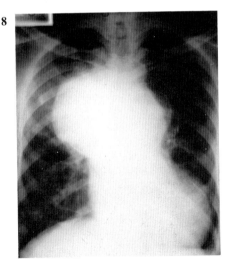

7 A 55-year-old man was admitted with lower sternal discomfort which started after a large meal and was associated with shortness of breath. Physical examination was normal.

(a) What does the ECG show?

(b) How would you manage him?

8 A 60-year-old man presents with a five month history of dysphagia and shortness of breath. On examination he is found to have a heart murmur.

(a) What are the abnormalities in the chest X-ray?

(b) How do you account for these abnormalities, his dysphagia and the murmur?

(c) What is the likely aetiology?

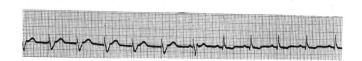

9 A 60-year-old man had a demand pacemaker implanted four years ago for intermittent complete AV block and dizziness; he now presents with rather similar symptoms.
(a) How do you account for the fact that he is in normal sinus rhythm without any pacing artefacts in the last part of the rhythm strip?
(b) Identify two abnormalities in the upper rhythm strip.
(c) What management for the patient do you suggest?

10 A woman presents with some upper epigastric pain. Initially admitted to exclude a myocardial infarct, on her second hospital day she developed these irritating lesions on her elbows.
(a) What might these lesions be?
(b) Where else might they be found?
(c) Why did she develop them?

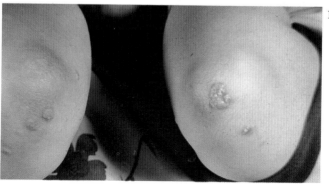

11

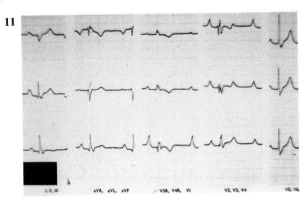

I, II, III	aVR, aVL, aVF	V5R, V4R, V1	V2, V3, V4	V5, V6

11 A 50-year-old woman with a long history of rather disabling recurrent palpitation and dizziness is known to have a heart murmur which is thought to be right-sided in origin. There is no clinical chamber hypertrophy. She has been thought to be mildly cyanosed in the past but this has become more pronounced recently. The only abnormality on X-ray is that of a large heart.

(a) Identify four abnormalities in the ECG.
(b) Why does she have episodes of palpitation and become so unwell with them?
(c) What factors contribute to her cyanosis?

12 A 45-year-old man is admitted with severe epigastric pain which started two hours before admission. He has never smoked and had no previous illnesses. He is still in some pain and has not yet received any analgesia. He is well perfused with a blood pressure of 130/85/85 mm Hg.

(a) Identify three abnormalities in the ECG.

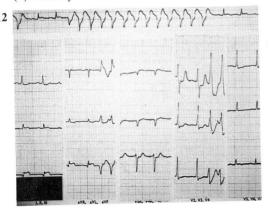

I, II, III	aVR, aVL, aVF	V3R, V4R, V1	V2, V3, V4	V5, V6, V7

(b) What treatment would you institute?
(c) Assuming he makes an uncomplicated recovery what is his likely percentage mortality rate over the ensuing twelve months?

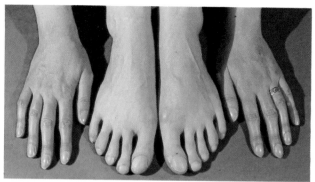

⁹ **13** A 45-year-old woman was found to have a heart murmur at the age of 15 years, when her parents noticed that her legs and arm were often a different colour compared with her friends. She was advised not to have any children. Her exercise tolerance is now quite limited by shortness of breath.
(a) What abnormalities do you note? How do you explain them?
(b) What complications of this condition might develop?
(c) Is there any treatment available?

14 A 64-year-old man who was 30 hours post operation had an emergency partial gastrectomy performed for a bleeding ulcer. He had been on digoxin for some years for heart failure but had not received any since before the operation. His immediate postoperative course had been satisfactory but he then at 2 am developed a tachycardia and dropped his blood pressure to 85/65/65 mm Hg.

(a) What are the main abnormalities?
(b) What investigation would you ask for at this time of night?
(c) How would you treat the problem?

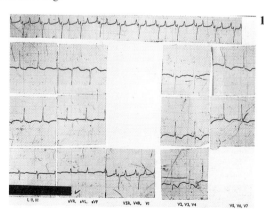

I, II, III   aVR, aVL, aVF   V3R, V4R, V1   V2, V3, V4   V5, V6, V7

15

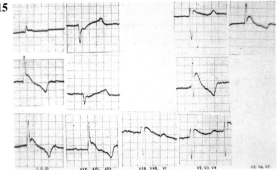

L.II, III   aVR, aVL, aVF   VSR, V4R, V1   V2, V3, V4   V5, V6, V7

15 A 67-year-old woman had a history of mild angina for several years. She was brought into the accident and emergency department in a confused state by her daughter. She was on no medication and was found to have a pulse of 40/min and a BP of 105/75/75 mm Hg.
(a) What are the main abnormalities in the ECG?
(b) What other information would you like to confirm your diagnosis?
(c) How would you treat this woman?
(d) What possible complications might you expect?

16 This is a simultaneous pressure tracing of the femoral artery and left ventricle with the ECG. The pressure range in mm Hg is included.
(a) What is the main abnormality?
(b) Which conditions might produce these pressure tracings?
(c) Is the abnormality mild, moderate or severe?

16

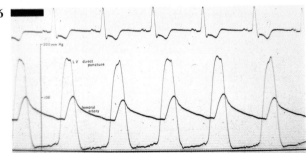

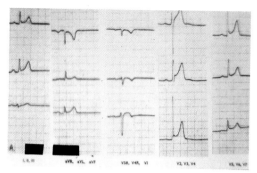

17 A 28-year-old Nigerian man presents with some left submammary pain which is made worse when he is under stress at work. There are no abnormalities on physical examination.
(a) How would you report this ECG? The patient is in sinus rhythm.
(b) Could this ECG be within normal limits?
(c) What measures could you use to demonstrate the fact that the tracing is normal?

18 A 45-year-old man was admitted with some right-sided chest pain associated with dizziness. No abnormalities were found on examination. He now presents with shortness of breath and central chest discomfort. His blood pressure has dropped to 95/70/70 mm Hg.
(a) What does the ECG show?
(b) What is the likely diagnosis and how might you confirm it?
(c) How would you treat this man now?
(d) How would you deal with his chest discomfort?

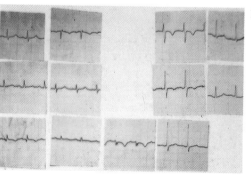

19

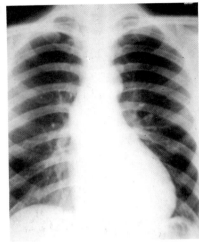

19 A 24-year-old patient had been referred because of a heart murmur, which had been discovered at an insurance medical examination.
(a) What abnormalities are present?
(b) What is the likely cause of his heart murmur?
(c) What advice does the patient need to be given?

20 A 34-year-old woman presented with some left-sided chest discomfort, shortness of breath and palpitation. On examination the heart was slightly irregular and there was a heart murmur that varied in intensity with posture.
(a) What abnormalities are present in the echocardiogram?
(b) What is the likely diagnosis and how do you explain the symptoms and signs?
(c) What is the natural history of the condition?

20

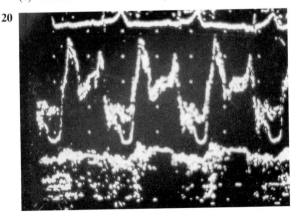

21 A 55-year-old woman who developed Raynaud's phenomenon ten years ago is now getting progressively more short of breath on exertion.

(a) What is the most likely diagnosis?

(b) What other symptom might she have?

(c) Why is she short of breath and how might her heart be implicated?

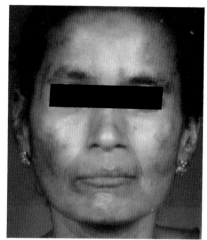

22 A 50-year-old man had a severe attack of indigestion about ten days previously. He now presents with shortness of breath on exertion and extreme fatigue.

(a) What abnormalities are there in the ECG?

(b) What is the most likely diagnosis?

(c) What is the mechanism of the shortness of breath?

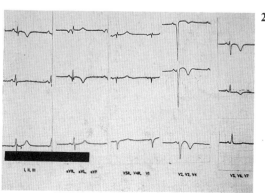

23

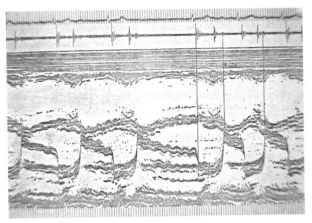

23 A man presents with a heart murmur and shortness of breath on exertion.
(a) What abnormalities are there on the echocardiogram?
(b) What is the likely diagnosis and how severe is it?
(c) What do the two lines from the echocardiogram correspond with on the phonocardiogram and how do you account for the abnormalities?

24

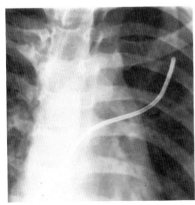

24 During a diagnostic cardiac catheterization the venous catheter which has been introduced via the femoral vein pursues the path displayed.
(a) What is the likely saturation of a blood sample taken from its tip?
(b) Name the vessel in which the tip of the vessel lies and describe the route the catheter took.
(c) What is the likely pressure in this vessel?

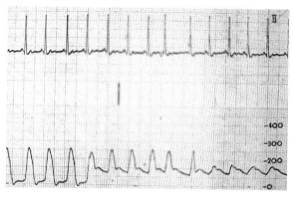

25 This withdrawal pressure tracing was recorded when the catheter was slowly drawn back from the left ventricle (starting on the left of the tracing) into the aorta. The ECG tracing at the top is to record the rhythm only. The patient had a heart murmur but was relatively asymptomatic.

(a) Describe the abnormality.

(b) Name two conditions that might produce this sort of withdrawal tracing.

26 A woman presenting with dizzy spells which occurred without any premonition was sometimes aware of her heart thumping during these spells.

(a) What does the ECG show?

(b) What simple procedure might you employ to determine the mechanism of the arrhythmia more accurately?

(c) What drug treatment might be most useful?

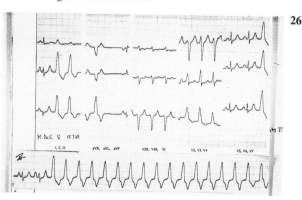

27 A man had a vein bypass graft for angina some five years ago; he now has little angina but needs treatment to keep him out of heart failure.

(a) What abnormalities are there on inspection of his chest?

(b) Name two cardiac drugs that may cause this problem.

(c) Apart from the aesthetic, are there any problems that may occur as a result of this problem?

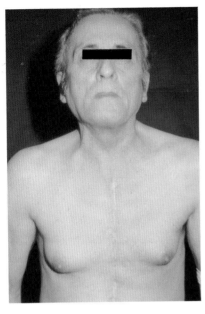

28 A 50-year-old woman presents with palpitation and a heart murmur. There is no heart failure and she is normotensive.

(a) What abnormality does she have in her hands?

(b) Why does she have a heart murmur?

(c) Is there a connection between these two problems? Is there an eponymous title for the condition and what is known of the aetiology?

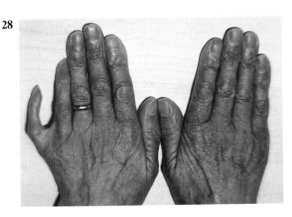

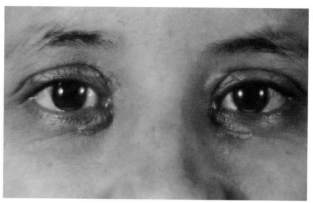

29 A 25-year-old woman from Kenya, of Indian parentage, is referred with the lesions around her eyes. She is otherwise asymptomatic.
(a) What is the composition of the lesions around her eyes?
(b) Are there any other abnormalities visible and what might their significance be?
(c) What measures should be taken after confirmation of the diagnosis?

30 On inflating the sphygmomanometer to 120 mm Hg the right hand of the patient rapidly adopted the displayed position.
(a) Why does the hand adopt this position?
(b) What associated abnormalities in the resting ECG might there be?
(c) Are there any described associations with this ECG abnormality?

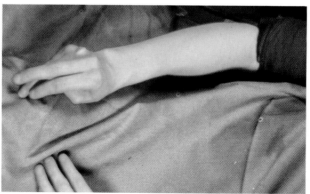

31

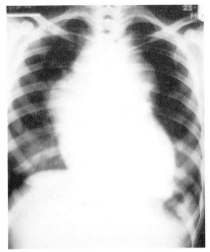

31 A 24-year-old woman presented with a short history of shortness of breath, sweating and some rather non-specific chest discomfort. On examination her venous pressure was raised and increased with inspiration; her pulse was 110/min and regular. Her blood pressure was 110/70/70 mm Hg and there was 30 mm Hg of paradox.

(a) What does the X-ray show?

(b) How do you explain her haemodynamic state?

(c) What is the likely aetiology?

(d) Why is the paradoxical pulse so called?

32

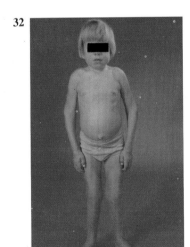

32 A nine-year-old boy is slightly mentally retarded. He has had a hunched back and rather swollen knees for some years. His abdomen has always been protuberant. Recently a heart murmur has been noted.

(a) What condition does this young boy have?

(b) What are the other characteristics of this condition?

(c) Why does he have a heart murmur?

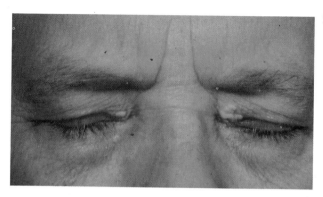

33 A 70-year-old woman was noted to have these lesions around her eyes some ten years ago; they have not changed in size in the interval. She is otherwise well.
(a) What are the lesions?
(b) What is their significance in this age group?
(c) If she had an arcus would this be of any significance?

34 A 64-year-old man had been known to have diabetes for at least ten years but had no symptoms of cardiac disease. He was due to have an aortic aneurysm operation.
(a) What abnormalities are there in the ECG?
(b) What conclusions can you reach about the extent of his heart problems?
(c) Are there any measures that you would advise in regard to the impending aneurysm operation?

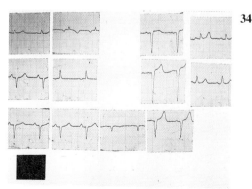

35

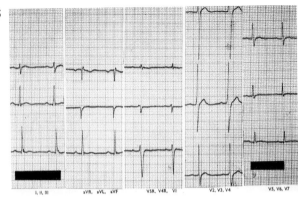

I, II, III   aVR, aVL, aVF   V5R, V4R, V1   V2, V3, V4   V5, V6, V7

35 A 36-year-old man presents with shortness of breath and had a very abnormal chest X-ray.
(a) How would you report the ECG?
(b) How could the abnormalities be related to his chest X-ray?

 36 A 43-year-old lady presents with a two year history of discomfort and swelling in her ankles and wrists. She was otherwise asymptomatic. On examination she was normotensive.
(a) What are the abnormalities on her hands?
(b) How do the hand abnormalities relate to her arthropathy?
(c) What is the cellular abnormality that accounts for her problems?

36

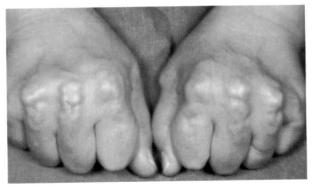

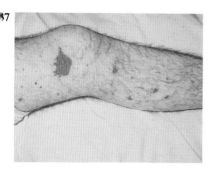
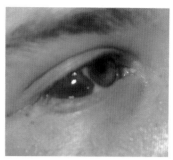

37, 38 A 20-year-old man presented with a fever and severe headache. His symptoms started twelve hours before admission. He had been previously well. His blood pressure on admission was 85/70/70 mm Hg. His pulse was 120/min. He rapidly became semi-comatosed. He had a skin rash over his trunk and more obviously over his legs. His eye was also abnormal.
(a) What condition do you think he has and how would you investigate and treat it?
(b) Why is the blood pressure so low and how would you manage it?
(c) Are there any other measures to be taken?

39 A 25-year-old man had a three day history of malaise and aches and pains together with a slight fever.
(a) What does the ECG show and what condition would you diagnose?
(b) Is there any other possibility that you would entertain?
(c) Is this always a benign condition? If not, what complications may occur?

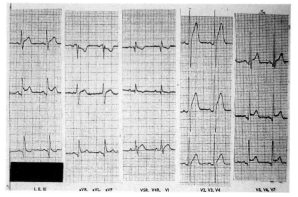

40

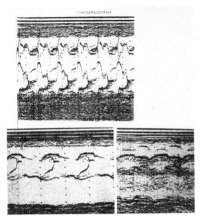

40 This M-mode echocardiogram was taken from a cyanosed neonate. The clinical diagnosis was that of congenital heart disease; there was no evidence of any lung disease. There are three views shown: the top is a view of the mitral and tricuspid valves; the lower left is a view of the aortic valve and left atrium; the lower right is a view of the pulmonary valve which is normal.

(a) What is the most striking abnormality?

(b) Why do you think the neonate is blue?

(c) Are there any other conditions associated with this lesion?

41 A 55-year-old man presenting with severe epigastric pain previously had a proven duodenal ulcer but had not had any symptoms from it for a number of years. When admitted his blood pressure was 80/60/60 mm Hg and he had a high venous pressure.

(a) What are the abnormalities?

(b) How would you manage the persistent hypotension?

(c) How do you explain the phenomenon of ST segment depression in this condition?

41

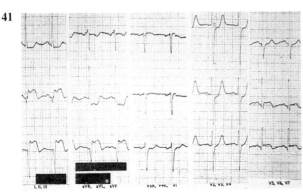

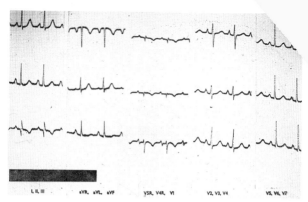

42 A 24-year-old woman was 32 weeks pregnant. She had been complaining of shortness of breath and palpitation. She had no chest discomfort. She had previously been in very good health.
(a) How would you report the ECG?
(b) What are the main changes in the cardiovascular system in pregnancy and how long do they last?
(c) What happens to these changes at delivery?

43 A 30-year-old patient, known to have a heart murmur for some years, had found her exercise tolerance to be markedly impaired. She had never been cyanosed but had fainted on exertion on several occasions. Her chest X-ray showed a normal sized heart with no evidence of any left to right shunt.
(a) What does the ECG show?
(b) What lesion might she have?
(c) What might be the management of such a patient?

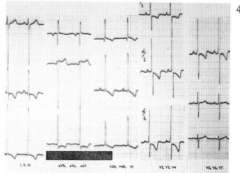

43

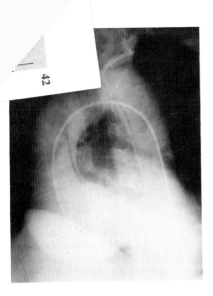

44 A patient had presented with central chest pain associated with sweating and shortness of breath. On examination he looked unwell; his BP was 95/80/75 mm Hg and pulse rate 120/min. A murmur was heard over the precordium.

(a) What does the aortogram show? (It is a left anterior oblique view.)

(b) How do you think he should be managed?

(c) What conditions predispose to the development of this problem?

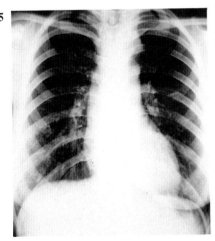

45 A 30-year-old woman is referred with a history of palpitation for many years. She was found to have a systolic murmur which was heard maximally in the aortic area and radiated to the neck; it was also well heard at the back. She had a blood pressure of 170/110/105 mm Hg. There was some evidence of LV hypertrophy clinically.

(a) What does the X-ray show?

(b) How do you fit the X-ray with the physical signs?

(c) Are there any other clinical associations that you need to consider?

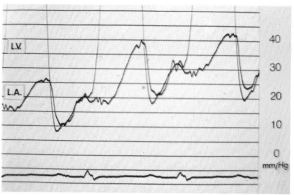

46 A pressure tracing of the left ventricle and left atrium, measured in mm Hg and ranged from 0 to 40 mm Hg. There is also an ECG tracing. The paper speed is 50 mm/sec. This patient has a long history of shortness of breath and has recently developed a heart murmur which has coincided with a deterioration in his symptoms.
(a) Identify three abnormalities in the tracings.
(b) What do you think the underlying problem is?
(c) How do you account for the heart murmur?

47 A seven-day-old neonate had severe respiratory problems which were related to heart failure. The child started to develop problems soon after birth. The child was not premature and had no heart murmurs. The mother had been ill with rather non-specific symptoms for the last month of the pregnancy.
(a) What does the ECG show?
(b) How do you account for the ECG and the heart failure at this age?
(c) What other causes of heart failure might you consider?

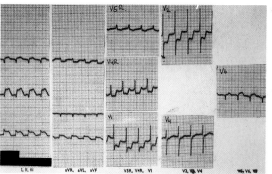

48 f. 312178

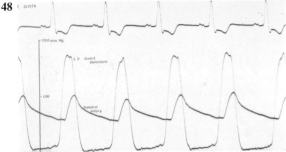

48 This tracing records the pressure in the left ventricle and the femoral artery simultaneously. The pressures are measured in mmHg and the scale is shown. There is also a simultaneously recorded ECG. The paper speed is 50 mm/sec. The patient was a 60-year-old man who presented with shortness of breath on exertion and was found to have a heart murmur.
(a) Name four conditions that might produce this record.
(b) How might you grade the severity of the lesion on the basis of the information given?
(c) In a normal person lying flat would the central aortic pressure usually be higher or lower than the femoral artery pressure?

49 This patient was entirely asymptomatic. She had a routine medical X-ray for work which was reported as being abnormal.
(a) What do you think the abnormalities are?
(b) How might you confirm the diagnosis?
(c) What complications are associated with this problem?

49

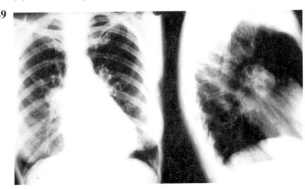

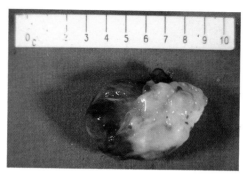

50 This mass was removed from the heart of a woman who presented with a stroke and was found to have a heart murmur.
(a) What do you think this mass is and where might it have been removed from?
(b) What other presentations are associated with this condition?
(c) How is the clinical suspicion of this condition best confirmed?

51 This valve was removed from a 55-year-old patient who was noted to have a heart murmur some ten years previously.
(a) What valve is it?
(b) What murmurs was the patient likely to have?
(c) What might a chest X-ray have shown in this patient before the valve was replaced?

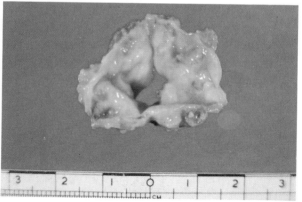

51

52

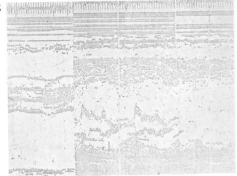

52 There are three views in this M-mode echocardiogram which was taken from a 65-year-old woman who was becoming increasingly symptomatic. She had been known to have a heart murmur for ten years. The physical signs had recently changed and suggested that her valve lesion was becoming more severe.
(a) Which valve is the main problem?
(b) Can any comment be made about her left ventricular function?
(c) Is there any other information that could be obtained by non-invasive means?

53 A 55-year-old man was admitted with central chest pain.
(a) How would you report this ECG?
(b) Assuming his pain has now settled and his blood pressure was only 85/70/70 mm Hg, what would you do?

53

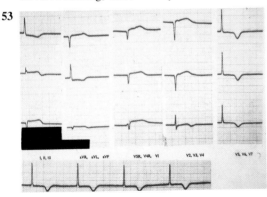

I, II, III   aVR, aVL, aVF   V5R, V4R, V1   V2, V3, V4   V5, V6, V7

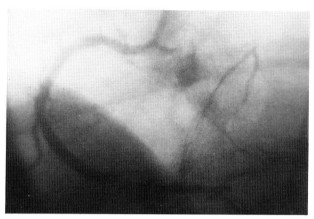

54 A right coronary arteriogram is taken in the left anterior oblique view. The patient had sustained an anterior infarct four years previously and was now suffering fairly severe angina on effort.
(a) Name five branches that are displayed in this arteriogram.
(b) Are there any abnormalities?
(c) What is the mortality risk from coronary arteriography?

55 This 24 hour ambulatory tape recording was from a patient with a history of syncopal attacks. Her resting ECG showed sinus rhythm with evidence of a bifascicular block.
(a) What does the displayed recording show?
(b) How should she be treated?
(c) What is the usual rhythm that causes death in this situation?

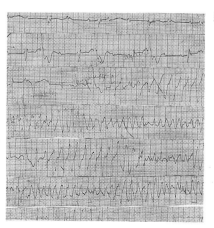

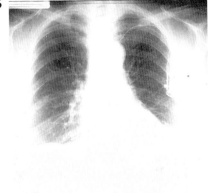

56 A 60-year-old woman presented with dizzy spells which proved to be due to transient AV block. She had a permanent pacemaker inserted.
(a) Where is the electrode tip placed and how?
(b) What precautions must a person with a permanent pacemaker observe?
(c) What might be a reasonable threshold to obtain at the time of insertion of the electrode and what is the power source?

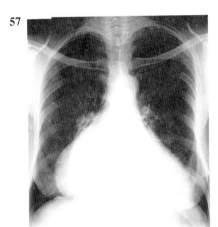

57 A 55-year-old woman who had surgery five years ago now presents with a high venous pressure, tender liver and oedema. Her lungs are clear.
(a) Identify four abnormalities in the X-ray.
(b) Are there any clues as to why she might have developed a high venous pressure and oedema?
(c) What added sounds is she likely to have from the mitral prosthetic valve?

58 This X-ray is taken some five years after the one shown in **57**. The patient has started to lose weight and has dysphagia.

(a) Is there any difference in the X-rays?

(b) What causes of dysphagia can occur in patients with mitral valve disease?

(c) How might the diagnosis be pursued in this patient?

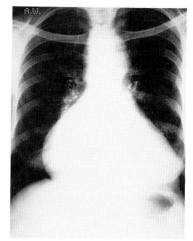

58

59 A man presents in casualty having been involved in a fracas outside a public house. He did not drink alcohol excessively himself. On examination the casualty officer found a wide pulse pressure and a BP of 150/65/60 mm Hg. There was a loud murmur which was well heard over the pulmonary area and adjacent area.

(a) How would you report this X-ray?

(b) How do you account for the murmur?

(c) What investigation would confirm the diagnosis and what would it show?

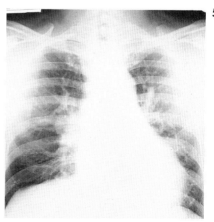

59

60

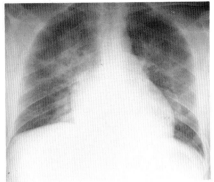

60 A 34-year-old man was admitted acutely ill with a BP of 80/65/65 mm Hg, a pulse rate of 130/min and a respiratory rate of 25/min. He had widespread crackles and wheezes and a gallop rhythm. He was peripherally cool and afebrile. He was acidotic; his arterial blood gases showed a pH of 7.02. His ECG showed a sinus tachycardia; there were some minor ST segment and T wave flattening only. He had been a heavy drinker until four years previously. He had a chest infection which started about five days before he was admitted. Prior to this he had been well and had a good exercise tolerance.
(a) What does the X-ray show?
(b) What is the likely cause for this problem?
(c) If he did not respond to diuretics, bicarbonate, digoxin, phlebotomy or inotropes, is there anything else you might consider?

61

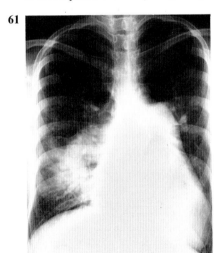

61 A 30-year-old woman was found to have a heart murmur at the age of five years. She is now cyanosed centrally; she has evidence of RV hypertrophy and a mid-systolic murmur in the pulmonary area. There is also a mid-diastolic murmur at the left sternal edge.
(a) What are the main abnormalities?
(b) What heart lesion does she have?
(c) Why is surgery not indicated?

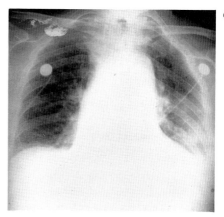

62 A 60-year-old man in a coronary care unit was known to have treated hypertension in the past. He developed severe central chest discomfort which was associated with sweating and shortness of breath. His BP was 250/140/135 mm Hg and his heart rate 120/min.
(a) How would you interpret the X-ray?
(b) What treatment would you introduce assuming that he was now free of pain?
(c) Are there any further investigations that you would request?

63 A 60-year-old man who had aortic valve disease gave a history of rheumatic fever as a child and was told that his valve was narrowed some 20 years ago. He also had a history of some dizzy spells and was taking aspirin for presumed vertebrobasilar insufficiency.
(a) What are the abnormalities in the ECG?
(b) How might this ECG relate to his symptoms?
(c) What treatment ought to be avoided?

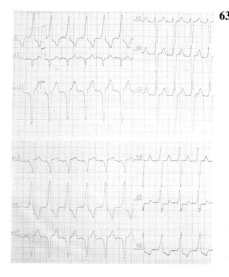

64

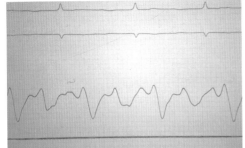

64 This tracing recorded at 50 mm/sec is of two ECG leads together with a jugular venous pulse recorded simultaneously. The patient had presented with a high venous pressure, a tender liver and peripheral oedema.
(a) Name the waves demonstrated in the recording and explain their genesis.
(b) Is there anything striking about the venous waveform?
(c) Suggest a possible diagnosis.

65

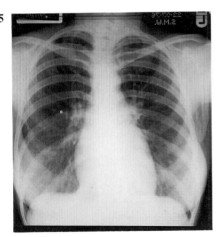

65 A 40-year-old woman presents with increasing shortness of breath, orthopnoea and tiredness. She is normotensive and has a heart murmur.
(a) How would you report this X-ray?
(b) Why is she short of breath?
(c) Name five complications of her condition.

66 A man in his 50s, who had rheumatic fever as a youth, has recently been getting more short of breath; his heart is getting larger and the murmurs more pronounced.
(a) Name two abnormalities in the echocardiogram.
(b) Are you able to determine what murmurs he has?
(c) Can you explain the pattern of movement in the mitral valve?

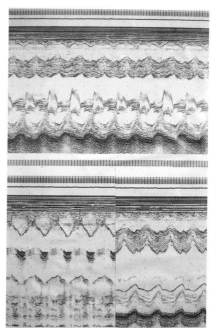

67 A patient who has collapsed in the street is brought in being resuscitated. There is no other history available.
(a) What rhythm is he in and how would you commence treatment?
(b) If he does not respond to your first measures, what might you do next?
(c) What conditions may predispose to this problem?

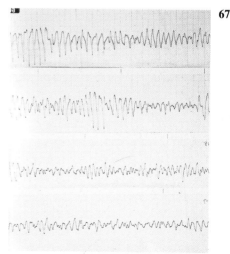

68

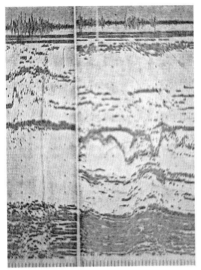

68 There are two views in this M-mode echocardiogram with a simultaneous phonocardiogram and ECG. The patient was mildly hypertensive and was referred by the GP for an opinion. A heart murmur was also commented upon.

(a) Name three abnormalities in the recording.

(b) Are you able to suggest a diagnosis?

(c) Is there any treatment that is required for this condition?

69, 70 At autopsy the mitral valve of this patient was found to be abnormal. No clinical diagnosis had been made prior to death. She had presented with a confusional state and a fever and died within two days of admission.

(a) What is the likely diagnosis?

(b) What is the prognosis for this condition in life?

(c) How is the diagnosis best made?

(d) How would you treat the condition and how would you know that the treatment was adequate?

69

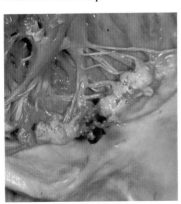
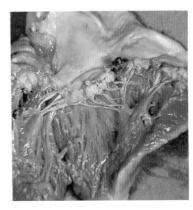

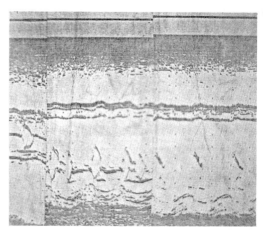

71 There are three views in this M-mode echocardiogram. The patient presented with a two year history of shortness of breath on exertion, orthopnoea and ankle swelling. He was normotensive. There was a very soft mid-systolic murmur at the apex, an elevated jugular venous pressure (JVP) and leg oedema.
(a) What are the main abnormalities?
(b) What is the likely diagnosis?
(c) What is the possible aetiology?

72 A 55-year-old patient presented to casualty with a chest infection and haemoptysis. A heart murmur was heard which had never previously been commented upon.
(a) What does the echo show?
(b) Is there any relationship with the chest infection?
(c) Is this study a satisfactory method of determining the severity of the heart problem?

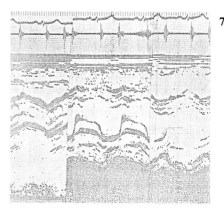

73

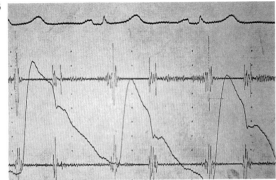

73 This is a simultaneous recording of the ECG, an indirect carotid artery tracing and two phonocardiographic channels (apical area above and pulmonary area below). The patient had been found to have a heart murmur when pregnant but was asymptomatic.
(a) Name four abnormalities.
(b) What information can you learn about the severity of this condition?
(c) When would you be most concerned about her heart condition as you look after her during the pregnancy?

74

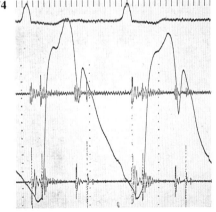

74 This is a simultaneous tracing of the ECG, an indirect carotid artery tracing and two phonocardiographic channels (pulmonary area above and mitral area below). The patient had heart surgery for valve trouble some three years previously and now has an improved exercise tolerance.
(a) Identify three abnormalities in the tracings.
(b) What type of valve surgery did the patient have?
(c) What complications are associated with these valves?

Site	Pressure (mmHg)	Saturation (%)
Right atrium	6	70
Right ventricle	110/6	78
Pulmonary artery	25/10	80
Left ventricle	120/10	94
Aorta	120/80	88
Left atrium	10	98

75 The data presented below was obtained at cardiac catheterization. The patient was a 22-year-old who had been told about a heart murmur at the age of four years but had not been followed up. He is now slightly cyanosed and has an impaired exercise tolerance.
(a) Name three abnormalities.
(b) What is the likely diagnosis?
(c) Name a number of complications of this condition.

76 This is a simultaneous tracing of the ECG, indirect carotid artery tracing and two phonocardiographic channels (aortic area above and mitral area below). The patient presents with a heart murmur but little in the way of symptoms.
(a) Name four abnormalities?
(b) What is the likely diagnosis?
(c) How could you assess the severity of the problem from the information given.

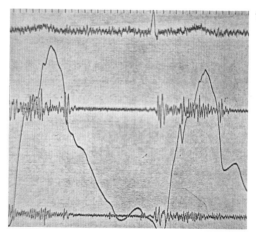

76

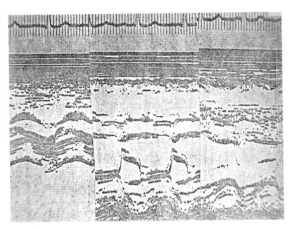

77 A 55-year-old patient had a history of rheumatic fever and was known to have a heart murmur.
(a) Identify the main abnormalities.
(b) What diagnosis seems likely?
(c) How severe is the problem?

78 The data shown below was obtained from cardiac catheterization. The patient was a 33-year-old complaining of increasing shortness of breath.
(a) Identify the abnormalities.
(b) What is the basis for the abnormalities?
(c) Suggest five possible aetiologies.

78

CATHETER DATA

Site	Pressure (mmHg)	Saturation (%)
Right atrium	5	68
Right ventricle	45/5	70
Pulmonary artery	45/25	70
PA wedge	24	—
Left ventricle	125/23	98
Aorta	125/85	97

79, 80 These two histological pictures of the myocardium of different magnification are from a patient who died suddenly whilst awaiting valve surgery.
(a) What is the abnormality seen?
(b) How might it relate to the patient's condition?
(c) How soon after this pathological event can changes be demonstrated in the laboratory?

Site	Pressure (mmHg)	Saturation (%)
Right atrium	3/0	70
Right ventricle	35/4	69
Pulmonary artery	35/15	85
PA wedge	9/5	—
Left ventricle	110/5	98
Aorta	110/80	98

81 The catheter data above was obtained from a 45-year-old man who was rather more short of breath over the past year than he had been previously. His GP arranged an X-ray as a result of which he was referred to you.
(a) What did the chest X-ray show?
(b) On which chamber of the heart does the load fall in this condition?
(c) How should it be treated?

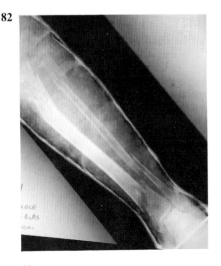

82 A 23-year-old man was involved in a road traffic accident. There was no suggestion of any head injury. After fixation of some of the broken bones, he was returned to the ward and made good progress for twelve hours. He then became rather confused and aggressive and was given some analgesia. An hour later he had a cardiac arrest.
(a) What possible causes for the arrest would you consider?
(b) What other complications might you be on the alert for after the resuscitation?

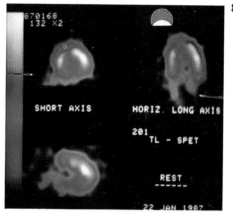

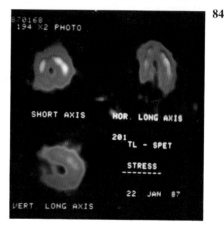

83, 84 A 45-year-old man had sustained a myocardial infarction some two years previously. He was now suffering from chest discomfort on exertion.

(a) Why is thallium used in these circumstances, rather than any other isotope, to determine the degree of reversible ischaemia?

(b) What does this scan show?

85 A 64-year-old patient presented with a transient stroke. The patient had been non-specifically unwell for a week before admission.

(a) How would you interpret the 2-D echocardiogram?

(b) How does it relate to the presentation?

(c) What should the further management be?

(d) Are there any long term problems that need be considered?

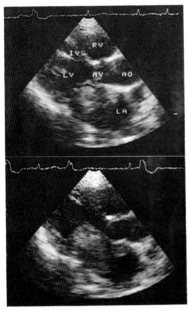

86 A 65-year-old patient was diagnosed as having mitral valve disease.

(a) How would you report this M-mode echocardiogram?

(b) What physical signs cause this condition to be confused with mitral valve disease?

(c) Name two limitations of M-mode echocardiography.

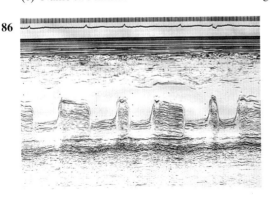

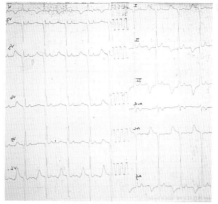

87 A 30-year-old woman presents with extreme shortness of breath on exertion. She is known to have had a heart murmur since a child.
(a) How would you report this ECG?
(b) What symptom might indicate a serious prognosis?

88 A 55-year-old man was admitted with lower sternal discomfort which started after a large meal and was associated with shortness of breath. Physical examination was normal.
(a) What does the ECG show?
(b) How would you manage him?

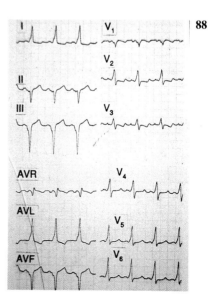

89

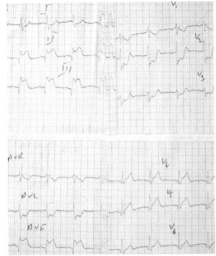

89 A 76-year-old man presented with severe chest and upper abdominal pain. His JVP was elevated, his lungs clear, his blood pressure was 90/70/70 mm Hg and he had a poor urine output.
(a) How would you report this ECG?
(b) What is the significance of the reciprocal changes?
(c) What is the first line of treatment for his blood pressure?

90 A 20-year-old man was admitted with chest pain. He had been complaining of tiredness for some weeks previously. He was normally very fit. On examination he was a tall, thin, fit-looking individual. Nothing abnormal was detected; his blood pressure was normal.

90

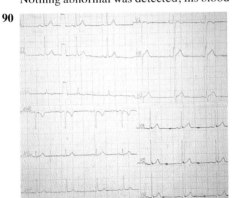

(a) How would you report the ECG?
(b) Does the ECG help in the making of a diagnosis in this instance?

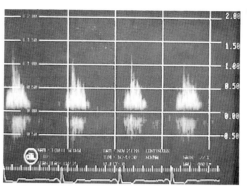

91 This continuous wave doppler study was performed from the suprasternal approach on a patient who had aortic stenosis due to previous rheumatic fever.
(a) What is the advantage of the continuous wave mode in this instance?
(b) What alternative to continuous wave doppler is there and what are its advantages?
(c) Can the severity of the valve lesion be estimated? If so how severe is the problem with this patient?

92 This continuous wave doppler using the apical approach was recorded from a patient with aortic valve disease.
(a) Can you comment on the significance of the waveforms?
(b) Can you quantify the severity of the lesions?
(c) Are there any other doppler techniques that can improve the diagnostic yield from this investigation?

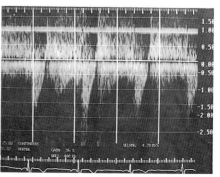

93

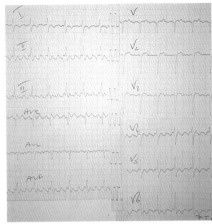

93 This patient was found to have a persistent tachycardia without an obvious cause.
(a) What is the cause of the tachycardia?
(b) Is there any way in which this arrhythmia could have been diagnosed at the bedside?
(c) Why is this rhythm often poorly tolerated?
(d) How would you treat it?

94 A 55-year-old woman came into casualty complaining of epigastric pain. Her BP was 85/75/70.

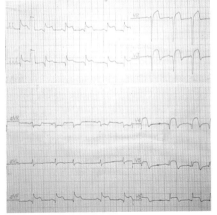

(a) What rhythm is she in?
(b) How might you prevent ventricular fibrillation?
(c) Why is she so hypotensive?

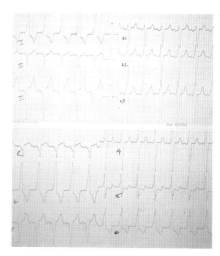

95 This ECG is from a man who comes into hospital with severe heart failure and a large heart. He had an aortic valve replacement two years previously.
(a) Comment on the ECG in regard to his failure.
(b) What treatment might you institute; he has only been on diuretics in the past.

96 A man who was known to be in atrial fibrillation in the past came in to hospital in gross heart failure with a BP of 75/50/50 and a heart rate of 170/min.
(a) What rhythm is he in?
(b) How would you treat it?
(c) If you were uncertain of the rhythm and wanted to confirm it, what might you do?

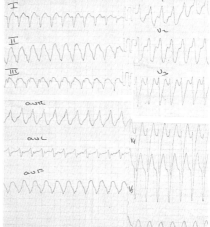

97

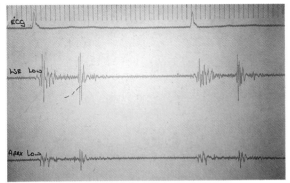

97 The simultaneous ECG and phonocardiogram was recorded from a woman who presented with shortness of breath.
(a) Name three abnormalities.
(b) Why might she be short of breath?
(c) What advantage does this type of recording have over the well trained human ear?

98 A 50-year-old woman who has a past history of rheumatic fever has been getting increasingly short of breath in the last few months.
(a) Which chamber of the heart is enlarged? Why might it be large?
(b) Which valve is affected? Explain its abnormal movements.
(c) Is there any abnormality of movement of the LV walls?

98

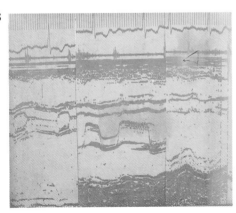

99 A 65-year-old woman presents with increasing tiredness, shortness of breath and fatigue.
(a) Which chambers of the heart can you confidently predict are large?
(b) Can you make any inference about pressures in the heart from the plain chest X-ray?

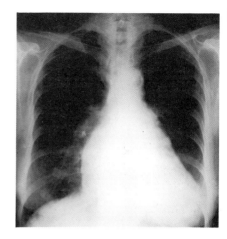

100 A patient was asymptomatic but was found to have a systolic murmur that had not been previously noted.
(a) How would you report the X-ray?
(b) Can you suggest the likely origin of her heart murmur?

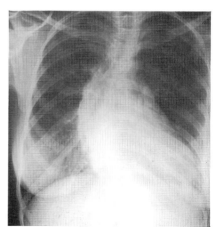

101

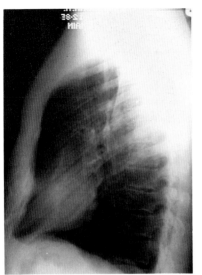

101 A 44-year-old man had an operation for a sternal depression for aesthetic reasons.

(a) As a result of the sternal depression, heart disease may be mistakenly diagnosed radiographically. Why?

(b) As a result of the sternal depression, heart disease may be mistakenly diagnosed clinically. How?

(c) As a result of the sternal depression, heart disease may be mistakenly diagnosed electrocardiographically. Why?

102 A 45-year-old Turkish man presents with a three week history of malaise, fever, cough and shortness of breath. On examination he was comfortable lying flat in bed; his blood pressure was 110/70/70 mm Hg; his pulse was 110/min; his respiratory rate was 19/min; his venous pressure was elevated 6 cm above the sternal angle and increased with inspiration; his temperature was 38.4 degrees.

(a) What does the X-ray show?

(b) How might you explain the physical signs?

(c) What other investigations might be useful?

102

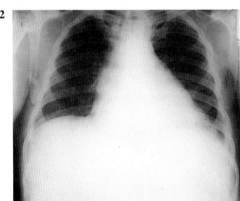

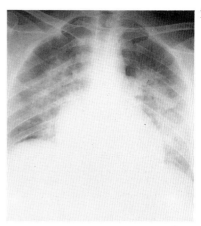

103 A previously fit 24-year-old presented with the rapid onset of shortness of breath over four to five hours. There was no preceding illness and no chest pain.
(a) What does the X-ray show?
(b) What conditions might lead to this presentation?
(c) How might this be treated?
(d) If the treatment specified does not work what condition might you consider?

104 A 34-year-old woman has rheumatic valvular disease but has few symptoms at the moment.
(a) On inspection of the X-ray what valvular problem do you think she might have?
(b) How might you determine the correct time for valve replacement?

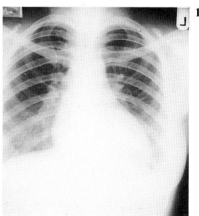

105

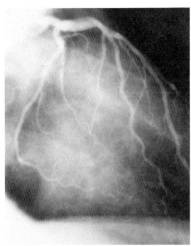

105 This is the right anterior oblique view of a coronary arteriogram of a patient.
(a) Which artery is it?
(b) Name five branches of this vessel.
(c) Does this vessel supply the conducting system of the heart? If so, does it supply it all or only part?
(d) Does this vessel supply any part of the interventricular septum? If so, which part?

106 A 33-year-old woman presented with palpitation and some shortness of breath. She had had some upper respiratory tract symptoms which were now improving. She was known to have had a normal chest X-ray six months previously.
(a) How would you report the X-ray?
(b) What do you think is the most likely diagnosis?
(c) Are there any dangers associated with this condition?

106

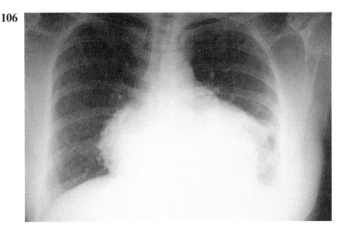

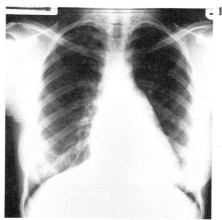

107 A woman has had a valve replacement.
(a) Which valve has been replaced?
(b) What sort of valve might be used in a young woman?
(c) Why might this type of valve be used particularly in a young woman?

108 A 55-year-old man had a valve replacement with a prosthetic Starr Edwards valve.
(a) Which valve has been replaced?
(b) What is the likely life of this sort of valve?
(c) What is the likely annual mortality from anticoagulation?

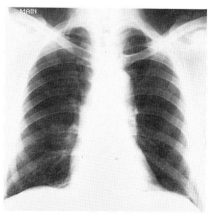

109

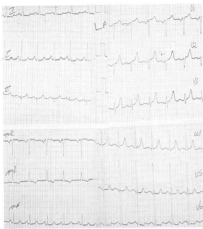

109 A 45-year-old man came into hospital with moderately severe heart failure. He was not on any treatment.
(a) How would you report this ECG?
(b) Can you comment on the left atrial pressure?

110 A 47-year-old man had some mild exercise-related chest discomfort. He had a normal resting ECG. This shows the ECG during an exercise test at stage 3 of the Bruce protocol.
(a) What abnormalities are demonstrated?
(b) How would you interpret these changes?
(c) What other information do you need about the exercise test?
(d) What is the risk of a maximal exercise stress test?

110

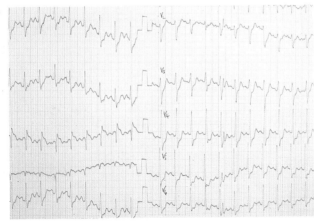

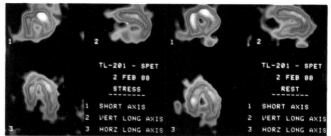

111 A 55-year-old man had exercise-related chest pain and was thought to have coronary artery disease.
(a) How would you report this thallium stress test?
(b) Which vessel is likely to be involved?
(c) In which ECG leads might ischaemic changes be seen?

112 A 45-year-old man had sustained a myocardial infarct some three years previously. He now presents with shortness of breath. His MUGA scan is shown.
(a) What comments would you make about the amplitude image?
(b) Is the phase image normal?
(c) The LV ejection fraction calculates out at 14 per cent; what comments do you have?
(d) What other information is contained within this study; how does it help in the management of the patient?

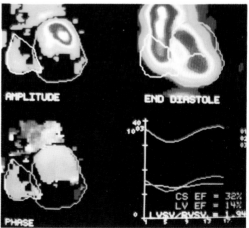

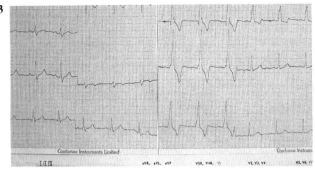

113 A woman had a pulmonary valvotomy performed ten years previously. She is asymptomatic but still has a loud systolic murmur in the pulmonary area.
(a) How do you report this ECG?
(b) Do you think she has a right ventricular hypertrophy?
(c) How will her second heart sound move?

114, 115 A 64-year-old woman presents with a history of occasional attacks of severe central chest discomfort radiating through to her back. Four years previously she had had her ascending aorta replaced because of aneurysmal dilatation; at this time she also had severe aortic regurgitation which was cured by the operation on the ascending aorta without a need to replace the valve. X-ray **114** was taken in 1984, **115** in 1988.

114

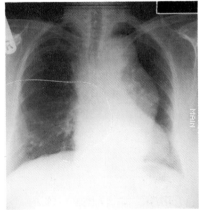

(a) What do these X-rays show?
(b) If surgery was advised, what would be the major morbidity risk; what sort of mortality risk might there be?
(c) What medical treatment might be helpful?
(d) What is the likely pathology underlying this condition?

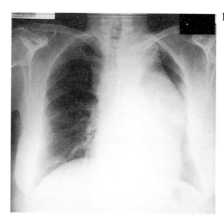

116 A 40-year-old woman presented with swollen ankles, distended abdomen and shortness of breath on exertion. These symptoms had been getting progressively worse over six months. On examination she had a normal blood pressure and a pulse rate of 95/min. She was comfortable lying in bed with one pillow. Her venous pressure was raised. There were no murmurs. Her abdomen was swollen and the liver was enlarged and tender. Cardiac catheter studies showed the following:

(a) Name the main abnormalities.
(b) What is likely cause of the problem?
(c) What is the best treatment?
(d) Why can she lie flat so easily?

116

Site	Pressure (mmHg)	Saturation (%)
Right atrium	a = 16, x = 8, v = 16, y = 5	70
Right ventricle	35/16	70
PA wedge	a = 17, x = 10, v = 16, y = 7	
Pulmonary artery	35/15	71
Left ventricle	120/17	98
Aorta	120/80	98

Site	Pressure (mmHg)	Saturation (%)
SVC		68
Right atrium	a = 12, x = 0, v = 6, y = 4	70
Right ventricle	175/6	70
Pulmonary artery	10/4	71
Left atrium	a = 8, x = 3, v = 10, y = 1	99
Left ventricle	120/7	98
Aorta	120/80	98

117 A 35-year-old woman presented with a minor cerebrovascular accident but made a full recovery after several weeks. She was found to have a heart murmur.
(a) Name the main abnormalities.
(b) What physical signs might she have?
(c) How might one explain the initial presentation?
(d) If she were to become cyanosed on exertion, what might be the reason?

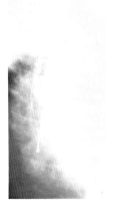

118 This patient was recovering from a myocardial infarction. The sleeve of an intravenous cannula had become sheared off from the hub and was sited in the right ventricle.
(a) What sort of catheter has been inserted?
(b) Why might there have been a need to insert this catheter?

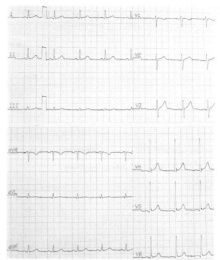

119 A 45-year-old patient had this routine preoperative ECG taken.
(a) How would you report this ECG?
(b) How valuable are routine preoperative ECGs?

120 A patient presented with a transient ischaemic episode and was found to have a heart murmur.
(a) What does the echocardiogram show?
(b) How do the findings on the echocardiogram relate to the phonocardiogram?
(c) What is the likely cause of the TIA?
(d) What treatment is indicated and when should it be instituted?

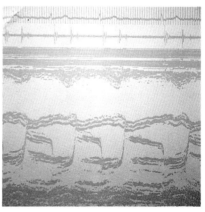

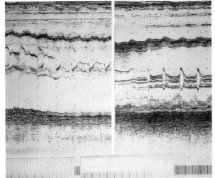

121 A 35-year-old man was admitted with severe shortness of breath, which had been developing over the preceding few weeks. When admitted he was in quite severe heart failure and had a systolic murmur.
(a) Identify seven abnormalities in these two views.
(b) What sort of pathological process may underlie this appearance?
(c) Why might he have a heart murmur?

122 A 70-year-old man came into hospital feeling very weak. He was found to have a haemoglobin of 6.8 G.
(a) How would you report the ECG that was taken?
(b) Might he have an abnormality of his second sound?

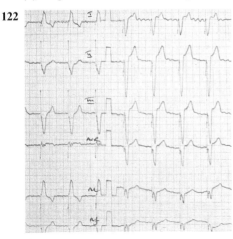

123 A 35-year-old woman presented with some epigastric pain lasting three hours and starting some 20 minutes after a large meal. She had a history of peptic pain in the past; the present pain was more severe than previously but in a similar position. When she was seen the pain had almost disappeared.

(a) How would you interpret the ECG?

(b) How would you treat her?

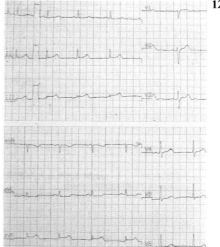

123

124 An 83-year-old man presented in the Accident and Emergency department with a history of a faint in the newsagents. He had previously been fit and well.

(a) Name four abnormalities in the ECG.

(b) How might his faint have been caused?

(c) What treatment does he need?

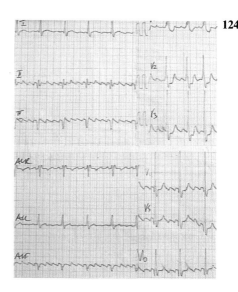

124

125

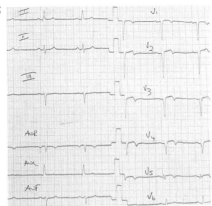

125 A 68-year-old patient was admitted to an orthopaedic ward for a hip replacement. Two weeks prior to admission he had a severe attack of indigestion.
(a) What does the ECG show?
(b) What advice would you give to the orthopaedic team?

126 A 34-year-old rather overweight woman who was a bus driver had a Public Service Vehicle licence. Physical examination was normal.
(a) How would you report this ECG?
(b) Can she continue to hold her PSV licence?

126

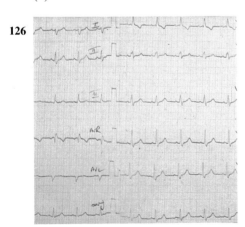

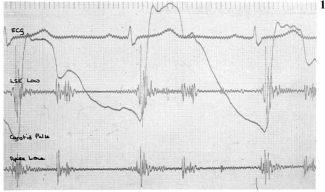

127 This is a simultaneous recording of the ECG, two phonocardiographic channels (LSE, low frequency and apex, low frequency) and the indirect carotid artery pulse. The recording speed is 50 mm/sec. The patient, a 55-year-old, has been told that there is a heart problem. She is asymptomatic.
(a) Can you identify three abnormalities?
(b) Can you suggest a possible diagnosis?
(c) Is there any other feature that you might expect to find if this patient's problem were a severe one?

128 A 55-year-old woman pre-sents with an atrial septal defect. The chambers are labelled.
(a) What abnormalities might be found in the 2-D echocardiogram?
(b) Why is this a superior investigation to the M-mode?
(c) Is there any major limitation to the 2-D as opposed to the M-mode?

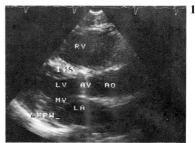

129

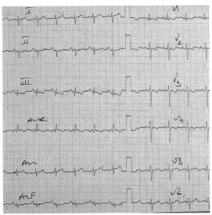

129 A 25-year-old woman presented with a history of two episodes of syncope on exertion. She was otherwise well. Physical examination was normal apart from a very short and soft systolic murmur at the left sternal edge and a loud second component of the second sound.

(a) How would you report this ECG?
(b) What information would you like to obtain from the chest X-ray?
(c) What other information would you particularly like to obtain from her?
(d) What information might be available if you were to perform cardiac catheterization?

130 The catheter data shown below were obtained from a young woman presenting with shortness of breath and syncope on exertion.
(a) Name three abnormalities.
(b) What diagnosis might you consider?
(c) What treatment is available for this condition?

130

Site	Pressure (mmHg)	Saturation (%)
SVC	—	69
IVC	—	71
Right atrium	a = 12, x = 4, v = 6, y = 4	70
Right ventricle	125/10	70
Pulmonary artery	125/85	71
PA wedge	a = 10, x = 5, v = 8, y = 3	
Left ventricle	120/7	98
Aorta	120/80	98

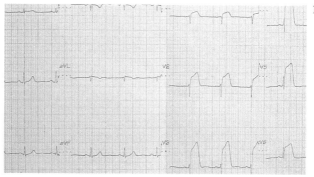

131 A 35-year-old man presented with severe chest pain radiating to his throat.
(a) What is the likely diagnosis?
(b) Could treatment cause the ECG to revert to normal?

132 This histological picture was taken from the coronary artery of a patient who had a history of angina for three years. He had collapsed and died whilst watching a football game.
(a) What does the picture show?
(b) What role does this play in the sudden death of this patient?
(c) Can this process be influenced to the patient's benefit?

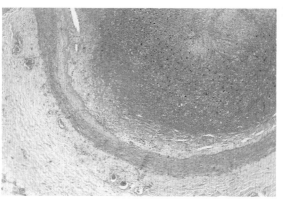

133

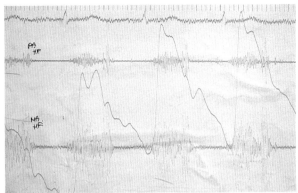

PA
HF

MA
HF

133 This simultaneous recording of the ECG, two phonocardiographic channels (the top one recording high frequency in the pulmonary area, and the lower tracing high frequency in the mitral area) and indirect carotid arterial tracing were taken from a lady who presented with a two year history of exercise-related shortness of breath. This had become much worse suddenly about two weeks before presentation. On examination she had no evidence of heart failure. She was normotensive and had a loud systolic murmur.
(a) Identify three abnormalities.
(b) What is the likely origin of the murmur?
(c) What is the likely aetiology?
(d) Why did she become suddenly worse?

134 A 60-year-old man had a history of rheumatic fever as a child, and had been known to have a heart murmur for the past ten years. He had become much more short of breath recently. The view of the mitral valve is reported to show fluttering of the mitral valve leaflet.

134

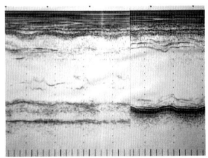

(a) What significance do you attach to the report of the mitral valve movements?
(b) What other abnormalities are present?
(c) Why has he become so short of breath?
(d) Should any action have been taken earlier?

135 A 65-year-old woman presents with a pneumonia and is found to have a heart murmur.

(a) What condition does she have?

(b) How might her heart problem be related to this condition?

(c) Are there any other heart problems associated?

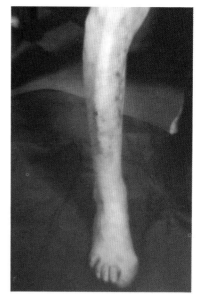

136 A patient presented 12 hours previously with severe central chest pain. The left venticular pressure is measured in mm Hg and the scale is on the left.

(a) Name two abnormalities.

(b) What is the most likely explanation of his chest pain?

(c) Explain anatomically how this condition can occur.

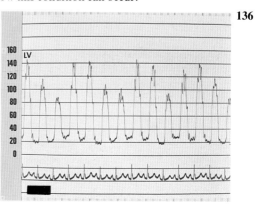

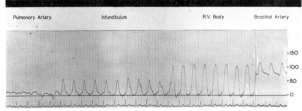

| Pulmonary Artery | Infundibulum | | R.V. Body | Brachial Artery |

137 A 13-year-old patient had been cyanosed for at least five years. The pressure is measured in mm Hg and the scale is shown. The recording is from the pulmonary artery to the right ventricle; it also shows the brachial artery pressure.
(a) Identify four abnormalities.
(b) Why is the patient cyanosed?
(c) What measures might the child take to intermittently improve the oxygenation?
(d) What treatment might now be offered the patient for this condition?

138 This M-mode echocardiogram was taken from a three-month-old cyanosed child. A heart murmur had been heard at birth and there was some cyanosis noted at this time. Over the next few weeks the cyanosis became more pronounced. The chambers of the heart are labelled.

138

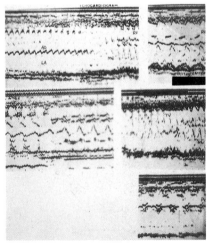

(a) Are all the valves present?
(b) Is there any abnormal relationship between the aorta and the rest of the heart?
(c) What is the diagnosis?

139 This patient with pulmonary stenosis was being catheterized from the right femoral vein. The blood drawn from the catheter in this site had a saturation of 97 per cent and the pressure was 100/7 mm Hg.

(a) Where is the tip of the catheter sited?

(b) How do you explain these findings?

(c) In what proportion of normal people is this manoeuvre possible?

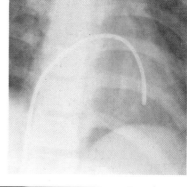

140 A 54-year-old woman presented with headaches.

(a) Name three abnormalities.

(b) What is the likely cause of these appearances?

(c) Prior to 1940 what was the likely prognosis?

(d) What is the likely prognosis nowadays?

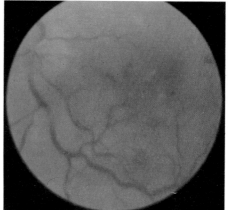

141 The selection of rhythm strips was taken from a 24 hour recording on a patient complaining of palpitation. A histogram of the heart rate is shown below.

(a) Name three abnormalities in the rhythm strip.

(b) What information does the histogram give?

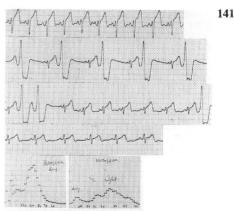

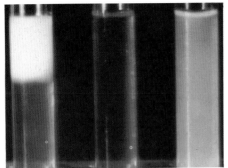

142 The three test tubes are samples taken from different patients in a fasting state. They all have lipid abnormalities.
(a) What is the likely lipid abnormality in the patient whose tube is on the left?
(b) What is the likely lipid abnormality in the patient whose tube is in the middle?
(c) What is the likely lipid abnormality in the patient whose tube is on the right?

143 A 35-year-old asymptomatic man had applied for life insurance. He was found to have a blood pressure of 150/95/95 mm Hg. Otherwise physical examination was thought to be normal.

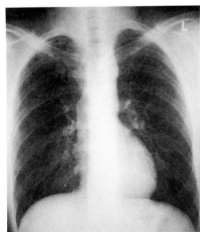

(a) How would you report the X-ray?
(b) Are there likely to be any associated abnormalities?
(c) What might the optic fundi show?
(d) What might happen if you exercise him?

144 A patient presents with tiredness and shortness of breath.
(a) What is the main abnormality and what is it due to?
(b) Name four complications of this abnormality.
(c) Name three means by which the diagnosis could be confirmed.

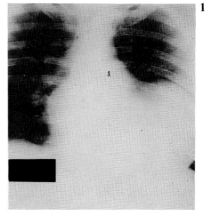

144

145 A 40-year-old man had developed mild aortic regurgitation 15 years previously. Over the ensuing years his regurgitation became progressively worse.
(a) Name two abnormalities.
(b) Can you suggest an aetiology for his aortic regurgitation?
(c) Can you give an explanation in pathological terms for your suggestion?
(d) What other clinical features might he have?
(e) Is there any predisposition to this condition?

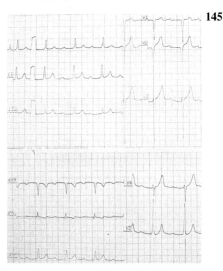

145

146

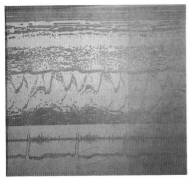

146 A man presented in the out-patients with a history of syncope associated with exertion. His primary care doctor had heard a heart murmur.

(a) Name two abnormalities.

(b) What is the diagnosis?

(c) What is the usual relationship of syncope to exertion in this condition.

(d) Is there any predisposition to develop this condition?

147

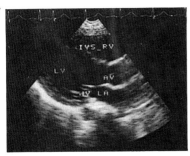

147 A 15-year-old boy presented with a high fever and a systolic murmur. The possibility of endocarditis on the mitral valve was raised on the request form.

(a) How would you report this echocardiogram?

(b) How would you advise about the possibility of endocarditis?

148

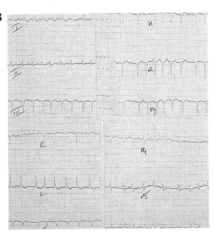

148 A 94-year-old woman was admitted with heart failure. She was on no treatment.

(a) How would you report this ECG?

(b) What treatment for her heart failure does she need?

149 A 66-year-old patient admitted from the Accident and Emergency department having been found collapsed at home. There was no other history available.

(a) Name three abnormalities.

(b) What is the most likely diagnosis?

(c) Give three reasons why the circulating volume of this patient might be low.

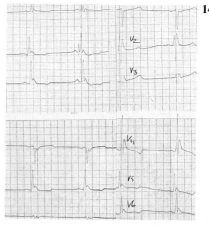

150 A 55-year-old woman had a history of intermittent shortness of breath.

(a) What isotopes are usually used for this investigation?

(b) Why is it necessary to perform both scans?

(c) What are the main abnormalities in this scan?

(d) If there was doubt about which was the perfusion and which the ventilation scan how might you tell?

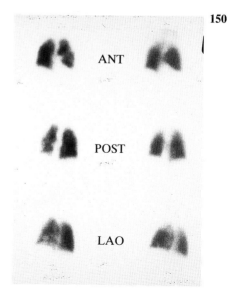

151

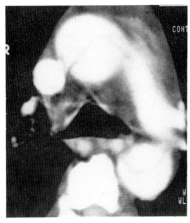

151 This CT scan taken at the level just below the aortic arch is from a patient who presented with chest pain. His ECG showed severe ischaemic changes.

(a) Why might the scan have been done?

(b) Can you identify any abnormality?

(c) What other information about this abnormality might you want?

(d) Why is the ECG ischaemic?

(e) What treatment is indicated?

152 This CT scan is taken at the level of the heart. The patient presented with chest pain and the ECG showed pronounced ischaemia.

(a) Identify the main abnormality.

(b) What is shown lying posterior to the ascending aorta?

(c) What are the two symmetrically placed structures which join the structure identified in (b)?

(d) What is the rounded structure lying on the left posterolateral aspect of the structure identified in (b)?

152

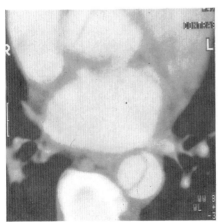

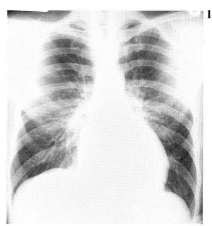

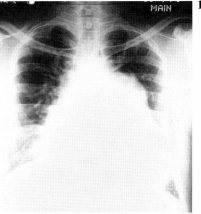

153 A 35-year-old homosexual presented with fatigue and shortness of breath. On examination he had a persistent sinus tachycardia and a normal blood pressure. He was apyrexial and had no heart murmurs. He had some crackles at both bases.

(a) What does the X-ray show?

(b) How might it relate to his symptoms?

(c) In what way could his sexual mores have played a part in causing his heart problem?

154 A 35-year-old man from Sri Lanka presents with shortness of breath and is found to have a loud heart murmur.

(a) What are the main abnormalities?

(b) What is the likely diagnosis?

(c) How do you think that this might be best treated?

(d) Are there any contraindications to the best form of treatment?

155

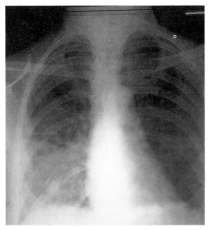

155 A 65-year-old woman was admitted to the ICU with progressively worsening shortness of breath. She was transferred from a medical ward where she was being treated for a stroke from which she was making a slow recovery. She was being fed with a nasogastric tube.
(a) Identify the main abnormalities.
(b) What is the likely cause of these changes?
(c) How is she best treated?

156 A 34-year-old woman presented with increasing shortness of breath, palpitation and ankle swelling. On examination she was found to be in mild heart failure and to have some heart murmurs.

156

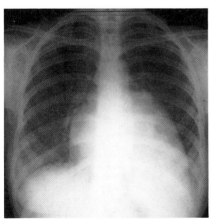

(a) Name three abnormalities
(b) Which chamber of the heart is the main culprit as regards her cardiomegaly?
(c) What is the likely aetiology of her problems?
(d) What choice in the type of valve replacement is there?

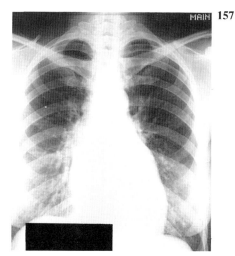

157, 158 These posteroanterior and lateral X-rays were taken from a patient who presented nine months previously with a history of shortness of breath and was found to be in atrial fibrillation and to have a heart murmur. She now presents with the sudden onset of a left-sided weakness.

(a) How would you report the posteroanterior film?

(b) How would you report the lateral film?

(c) Is there any gut problem that may be associated with this patient's problems?

(d) How would you now manage her stroke?

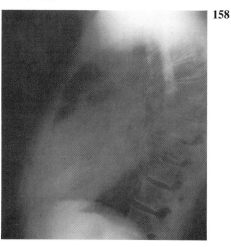

159

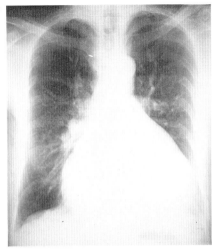

159 A 62-year-old man admitted with dyspepsia was found to have a heart murmur. He admitted to increasing shortness of breath over the preceding two years. When in hospital for a hernia repair four years previously no comment was made about any heart murmur. He now has a displaced apex beat, a systolic thrill and a systolic murmur.
(a) Identify three abnormalities.
(b) What is the likely problem with this man and what is the aetiology?
(c) How might the diagnosis be confirmed?
(d) How is he best managed?

160

160 A 76-year-old woman with hypertension presents with dizzy spells.
(a) Name three abnormalities.
(b) What is the likely cause of her dizzy spells?
(c) How would you treat her?

161 A man was referred with an irregular pulse and some chest discomfort.
(a) How would you report the ECG?
(b) How do you account for the abnormalities?

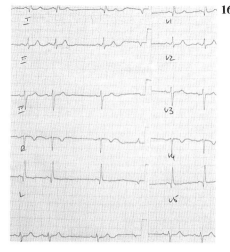

162 A 60-year-old man in the Accident and Emergency department is very short of breath and has mild left-sided chest discomfort.
(a) How would you interpret the ECG?
(b) What action might you take?

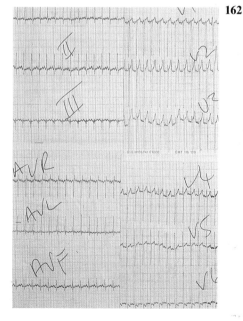

163

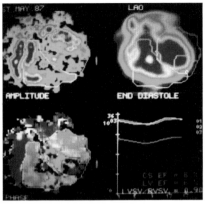

163 The radioisotope study was performed on this patient because he complained of severe shortness of breath which was sometimes associated with exertional chest discomfort. He had become very limited by his symptoms in spite of drug therapy.

(a) What radioisotope study has been performed?
(b) Can you explain the principle of it.
(c) Are there any conditions of the patient which make this study virtually impossible?
(d) In which circumstances is this investigation particularly useful?
(e) What does this scan show?

164

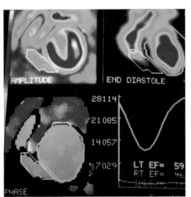

164 A woman presenting with angina was found to have a systolic murmur.

(a) What does the short axis view of the aortic valve show?
(b) What does the long axis view show?
(c) What is the likely explanation of her problems?
(d) Can we gain any more information about the severity of the condition by non-invasive means? Name three such means.

165

165 This MUGA scan was performed on a patient complaining of increasing shortness of breath on exertion.
(a) Explain the terms 'phase' and 'amplitude' which are the titles for the two pictures on the left.
(b) The ejection fraction is calculated as 59 per cent. Is this normal?
(c) What comments do you have about this study?

166 This patient presented with a slow regular bradycardia. These three leads were simultaneously recorded; the top recording is from an oesophageal lead at 30 cm from the mouth. The middle tracing is V1 and the lower V4.

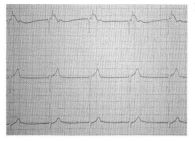

(a) What is the rhythm?
(b) Could you diagnose this clinically at the bedside?
(c) What is the virtue of the oesophageal lead?

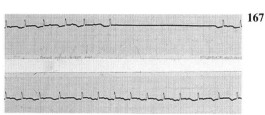

167 This continuous rhythm strip of lead I was taken from a patient who was complaining of dizzy spells and who had collapsed on one occasion.
(a) What rhythms are present?
(b) How might you treat this patient?
(c) What sort of disease process is present?

168 A 25-year-old woman had collapsed at home. There was no past history of heart disease.

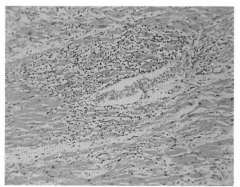

(a) What abnormalities are present in this histological section of her heart?
(b) What is the likely diagnosis?
(c) How common is this problem?
(d) What advice can be given to patients with this condition to reduce the risk of death?

169

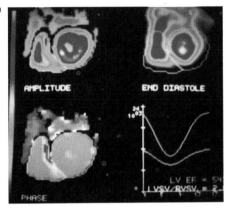

AMPLITUDE

END DIASTOLE

PHASE

LV EF = 54
LVSV/RVSV = 2.

169 This MUGA scan was obtained from a patient who presented with heart failure and was found to have a murmur of aortic regurgitation.
(a) What does the term MUGA mean?
(b) What isotope is usually used?
(c) How do you account for the LVSV/RVSV of 2.89? (LVSV = left ventricular stroke volume etc).
(d) Can you make any judgement about LV function?

170 A 55-year-old man had a history of angina. He had sustained an inferior myocardial infarct some five years previously. He managed to reach stage 2 of the Bruce protocol but had to stop because of the onset of his central chest discomfort. His blood pressure response was normal.
(a) What is a normal blood pressure response in these circumstances?
(b) What is the likely distribution of his significant coronary artery lesions?
(c) How specific and how sensitive is this investigation?
(d) What other factor influences the sensitivity and specificity?

170

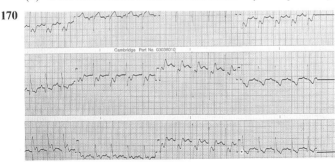

Cambridge Part No. 03038010

171 A 50-year-old patient presented with angina of effort and dizziness after exertion. A systolic murmur was found with a normal second sound.

(a) Name four abnormalities in the recording.

(b) What is the likely diagnosis?

(c) Are the symptoms described typical or atypical; explain your answer.

(d) Why might the patient die and how might it be prevented?

(e) Should the family be screened?

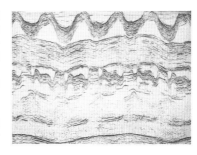

172, 173 A patient presents with the signs of a bicuspid aortic valve and mild hypertension.

(a) What condition does the patient have?

(b) Why is surgery usually recommended?

(c) What is the particular risk of surgery in this condition?

(d) What physical signs is the patient likely to have?

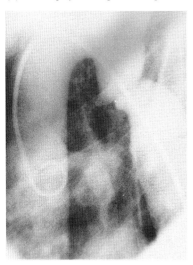
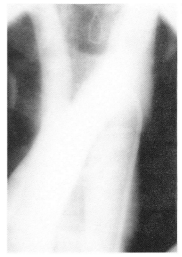

174

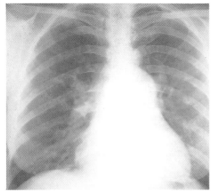

174 A 65-year-old woman has had a murmur for a number of years. She has noted increasing shortness of breath in the past year or two.
(a) What are the main abnormalities?
(b) What is the likely diagnosis?
(c) How severe is the lesion?
(d) How might you determine the advisability of surgery?

175 A 20-year-old woman presented with haemoptysis, shortness of breath and palpitation. She was also three months pregnant. She had a heart murmur and a thrill.
(a) How would you report this film?
(b) Why did she have a haemoptysis?
(c) What is the most difficult time haemodynamically for her during her pregnancy?
(d) If she needed heart surgery during the pregnancy, when should it be done?

175

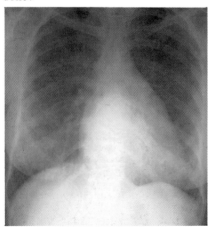

176 An 86-year-old woman had rheumatic fever as a child and is known to have valvular disease.

(a) How would you report this X-ray?

(b) Which chambers of the heart are particularly enlarged?

(c) Do these enlarged chambers confer any advantage to the patient?

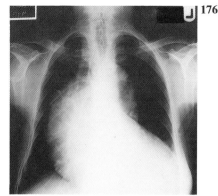

176

177 This patient was referred for an ECG because of palpitation; the referring doctor also mentioned a loud P2.

(a) How would you report the ECG?

(b) Why is P2 loud?

(c) What further measure would you like to take?

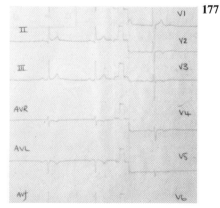

177

178 A 44-year-old man was found to have a heart murmur which was maximal in the aortic area.

(a) What abnormalities are present?

(b) What is the likely diagnosis?

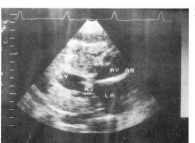

178

179

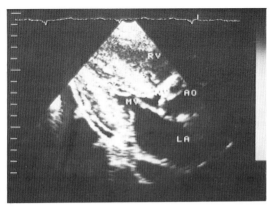

179 A 72-year-old man presents with high venous pressure and a gallop rhythm.
(a) What view is displayed?
(b) Name four abnormalities.
(c) Why might the myocardium appear so echogenic?

180 A 27-year-old drug addict presented with a fever, cough and sputum expectoration. She also had withdrawal symptoms.
(a) How would you report the X-ray?
(b) Why does she have this abnormal X-ray?
(c) If the presenting condition recurs after treatment, what diagnosis would you consider?

180

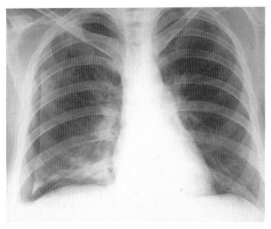

ANSWERS

1 (a) Saphenous vein bypass graft. The internal mammary artery is increasingly being used as an alternative. It may give better symptom relief for a longer period of time although the operation itself is technically more difficult.
(b) The mortality rate should be between 1 and 3 per cent. It is approximately twice as high in women.
(c) Approximately 50 per cent of patients have angina again after five years which progressively rises to about 80 per cent after ten years; these figures are better if the internal mammary graft has been used.

2 (a) Complete AV block (third degree AV block) with a high ventricular focus; this is consistent with a congenital aetiology.
(b) The H deflection represents depolarization of the bundle of His and the V deflection the depolarization of the ventricles.
(c) The H-V interval can be useful in helping to predict the progression from first or second degree AV block to complete heart block; it can also be useful in someone who is having symptoms of syncope but whose ECG is unhelpful.

3 (a) The intimal tear of an aortic dissection occurring just above the aortic valve.
(b) The dissection can track down towards, and then along a coronary artery. This may cause myocardial ischaemia or infarction, and ventricular fibrillation.
(c) Marfan's syndrome and systemic hypertension predispose to aortic dissection.

4 (a) High pulmonary artery wedge pressure and a diastolic pressure difference across the mitral valve. There is also a slow Y descent. This patient has severe mitral stenosis.
(b) Systemic embolization is a significant risk; the fact that the patient is in sinus rhythm does not remove the likelihood of embolisation. Atrial fibrillation can be a very serious problem for a patient with this degree of mitral stenosis. Pulmonary oedema may then develop and can sometimes result in death.
(c) The pulmonary artery pressure will be elevated; the extent of this elevation will depend on the pulmonary vascular resistance. It will be at least 35/20 mmHg but may be as high as 85/55 mmHg.

5 (a) The right coronary artery.
(b) It runs in the atrioventricular groove around to the back of the heart where, in about 80 per cent of individuals, it gives off the branch to the atrioventricular node and the posterior descending coronary artery.
(c) The main branches are: the conus artery; the right ventricular or acute marginal branch; the atrioventricular node branch; the posterior descending artery (in about 80 per cent of individuals) posterior ventricular branches.

6 (a) Very large proximal pulmonary arteries to each zone of the lung (ie plethora); calcification within the pulmonary arteries; rapid change in the calibre of the pulmonary arteries rather than a smooth tapering (ie pruning); large heart.

(b) A left to right shunt in which pulmonary arterial hypertension has developed. The development of cyanosis means that the shunt has now begun to reverse. The only lesion that produces such large pulmonary arteries and a large heart is an atrial septal defect.

(c) There is now no place for surgery. Indeed an operation might actually shorten her life. The treatment therefore is tailored for the complications such as polycythaemia or heart failure.

7 (a) A delta wave; a short PR interval; repolarization abnormalities (abnormal ST segments and T waves); Q waves in III and aVF.

(b) The Wolff-Parkinson-White syndrome is an intermittent phenomenon.

(c) A reciprocating atrial tachycardia; the impulses pass anterogradely down through the AV node and retrogradely back up the accessory bundle. These arrhythmias are usually benign and of nuisance value only. There are a small group of patients who develop atrial fibrillation; this is of more serious significance and may be associated with the development of ventricular fibrillation and sudden death. This group of patients need further electrophysiological investigations and may require ablation of the accessory bundle or long term anti-arrhythmic drug treatment.

8 (a) An enlarged heart; a large, smooth mediastinal mass; calcification within the mediastinal mass; opacification of the right upper zone of the lung.

(b) The mass is an aneurysm in the ascending aorta and also involving the arch; it is causing pressure on the oesophagus and on the right upper lobe bronchus. It has also caused widening of the aortic root thus causing aortic regurgitation.

(c) Syphilis.

9 (a) His AV block is intermittent; the pacemaker is on demand and his own complexes will therefore suppress any pacemaker impulses.

(b) A very fast pacing rate and a failure to capture (the third and fourth pacing artefacts do not capture the ventricle).

(c) The pacemaker needs to be changed.

10 (a) Eruptive xanthomata.

(b) On the buttocks.

(c) She probably has pancreatitis and resulting high lipid levels.

11 (a) Marked right axis deviation; very large P waves suggesting right atrial enlargement; right bundle branch block; long PR interval.

(b) The palpitation is due to atrial tachyarrhythmias. Her atrial transport is very important to maintain right ventricular output; without it she becomes very unwell.

(c) With a high right atrial pressure due to her Ebstein's anomaly, she will shunt right to left through a patent foramen ovale or an atrial septal defect. The anomaly is characterized by atrialization of part of the right ventricle; the remaining right ventricle may itself be abnormal. A large part of the output from the right side of the heart is therefore dependent on right atrial contraction.

12 (a) Changes of an acute inferior infarction namely ST segment elevation in II, III, aVF with reciprocal ST segment depression in I, aVL, V1, V2; episodes of ventricular tachycardia; T wave changes in the lateral praecordial leads.
(b) The main treatment to be introduced immediately is: (i) aspirin chewed, swallowed or given intravenously; (ii) a thrombolytic agent intravenously; (iii) pain relief in the form of an intravenous opiate; (iv) an anti-arrhythmic would only be introduced if the ventricular tachycardia persisted after the first two measures and was also causing haemodynamic disturbance.
(c) 2-4 per cent per annum for a man of this age who does not smoke and who has a good ejection fraction after his infarct.

13 (a) She has differential cyanosis; her left hand and both legs are cyanosed whilst her right hand is normal. The reversed shunt of a patent ductus usually allows desaturated blood to enter the aorta just proximal to the origin of the left subclavian artery; it can sometimes enter just distal in which case the left arm will be a normal colour.
(b) Polycythaemia with its adverse effect on viscosity leading to thrombotic problems; hyperuricaemia; paradoxical emboli; right heart failure; cerebral emboli.
(c) Once the shunt has reversed there is no place for closure of the duct. Certain drugs have been tried to attempt to reduce the pulmonary vascular resistance; they do not usually have a sustained effect although occasionally they can be dramatic in an individual. The only other treatment possibility is that of heart and lung transplantation.

14 (a) An atrial tachycardia with a 2:1 AV block, widespread ST segment and T wave abnormalities together with U waves.
(b) A serum potassium, which was 2.3 mmol/l.
(c) An infusion of 60 mmol of potassium in 500 ccs of saline corrected the arrhythmia and improved the blood pressure.

15 (a) J waves; a bradycardia; shiver waves; a long QT interval; idioventricular rhythm.
(b) A rectal temperature, which was 32^0C.
(c) Very gentle and slow rewarming, intravenous fluids and treatment of any precipitating factor such as a pneumonia, myocardial infarct, hypothyroidism.
(d) Arrhythmias; hypovolaemia; pancreatitis; hypokalaemia.

16 (a) A pressure difference in systole between the left ventricle and the femoral artery.
(b) Aortic valve stenosis; subvalve stenosis; supravalve stenosis; coarctation of the aorta.
(c) There is about 80 mmHg difference between the left ventricle and the femoral artery which is severe. The actual problem in this instance was aortic valve stenosis; an aortic valve replacement was subsequently performed.

17 (a) Sinus rhythm with a normal PR interval; normal QRS axis; raised ST segments in leads I, V2-V6, this is maximal in V3-V5 and is associated with a high take off.
(b) Yes. It is a normal variant. It is found in males in all races and is becoming more recognized with the increased use of ECGs. It is extremely rare in women.

(c) Exercise will bring ST segment down to the isoelectric line. Alternatively a small dose of intravenous atropine can be used which will produce the same effect. It is important, of course, to be certain that the ST segment abnormality does not represent some more sinister pathology before embarking on these measures.

18 (a) Sinus tachycardia with evidence of acute right heart strain; this is manifest by an S1, Q3, T3 pattern together with a partial right bundle branch block and T wave changes in the right precordial leads.
(b) Acute major pulmonary embolus. If there is doubt about the diagnosis on clinical grounds, the definitive test is a pulmonary angiogram.
(c) The choice of drug lies between heparin, streptokinase and a tissue plasminogen activator (tPA). tPA cannot yet be considered for general clinical use for this condition. There are problems associated with widespread bleeding with the use of streptokinase. Most patients do very well with heparin. Surgery has a very small role; it can be used if the patient fails to respond to treatment. Good medical treatment also involves the maintenance of a high filling pressure for the right ventricle,
(d) Drugs that cause venodilatation must be avoided; thus the opiates are contraindicated. Chest discomfort is best dealt with by the use of drugs such as aspirin, paracetamol or dihydrocodeine.

19 (a) The ascending aorta is very prominent. It is difficult to be certain whether there is cardiomegaly because the right side of the chest has been cut off; however the shape of the heart suggests that there is an increase in the size of the ventricular cavity.
(b) At this age the most likely diagnosis is a congenital bicuspid aortic valve; the combination of the prominent ascending aorta and the shape and size of the ventricular cavity suggests that the valve is both stenotic and incompetent.
(c) There are three main areas where advice is required: (i) the haemodynamic effect of the lesions must be assessed and advice given in regard to lifestyle, follow up intervals and need for further investigations; (ii) advice about the importance of antibiotic cover for any potentially septic procedures; (iii) the condition is inherited as an autosomal dominant; there is a need to screen the first degree relatives.

20 (a) The M-mode echocardiogram shows a wide amplitude of movement of the mitral valve. There is a prolapse or posterior displacement of the leaflet(s) in systole; this movement can vary both in amplitude and duration in the same patient at different times.
(b) Mitral valve prolapse. It is important to exclude the possibility of an underlying cardiomyopathy; the echocardiogram is a useful investigation for this condition. The prolapse is caused by myxomatous degeneration of the mitral valve and can be associated with chest pain and arrhythmias; historically it is therefore very important to exclude the possibility of myocardial ischaemia. The murmur can vary markedly with different postures and may be inaudible at times; postures that increase LV wall tension will increase the intensity of the murmur.
(c) On the basis that the condition has been shown to be an isolated mitral valve abnormality due to myxomatous degeneration, the condition is almost always benign. Antibiotic cover needs to be given for potentially septic procedures.

21 (a) Scleroderma. The history in conjunction with the puckering around her mouth and the telangiectatic spots on her nose and cheek make this diagnosis very likely.

(b) Difficulty in swallowing.

(c) The most likely cause of her shortness of breath is associated pulmonary fibrosis. This can affect the heart; sometimes pulmonary hypertension can develop without much lung involvement. The heart can also be involved by a vasculitis which may produce fibrotic changes in the myocardium; pericarditis is also fairly common. The disease virtually never affects the heart valves.

22 (a) There are deep Q waves in the anteroseptal leads associated with T wave inversion in I, aVL and V2-V5. There is also poor R wave progression across the precordial leads.

(b) An acute anteroseptal myocardial infarction occurring at the time of his severe indigestion.

(c) A raised diastolic pressure in the left ventricle will result from the extensive heart attack. The left atrial pressure will rise as a result causing pulmonary venous hypertension and stiffer lungs will ensue.

23 (a) A thickened anterior leaflet which closes very slowly producing a reduced E-F slope; the posterior leaflet is not well seen but is probably not moving very much; the mitral valve ring is also very thickened.

(b) Mitral valve stenosis due to rheumatic heart disease. It is very difficult to judge the severity from the M-mode echocardiogram. The E-F slope and the relative slopes of the anterior and posterior leaflets have been used but do not give a very accurate estimate. The echocardiogram gives structural information and any attempt to gain haemodynamic data from it is fraught with difficulty. Echo/doppler gives additional information about flow.

(c) One line corresponds to the opening snap and the other to the mitral valve closure which may be loud. The latter occurs because the valve is snapped shut by the very rapidly rising LV pressure which overcomes the elevated left atrial pressure. The opening snap occurs when the LV diastolic pressure falls below the elevated LA pressure.

24 (a) 96-99 per cent saturation.

(b) Left upper pulmonary vein. IVC-> RA-> LA-> PV; the passage through the atrial septum is either through a patent foramen ovale or an atrial septal defect.

(c) It will be the same as the left atrial pressure which in the normal person is 8-12 mmHg.

25 (a) There is a pressure difference within the aorta; the catheter is withdrawn from the LV (with a low diastolic pressure) into the aorta; there is no difference in the systolic pressure between LV and aorta (ie there is no aortic valve stenosis). However on withdrawing a little further into the aorta there is a pressure drop of about 70 mmHg.

(b) This could occur in a supravalve aortic stenosis or in a coarctation of the aorta.

26 (a) The most striking abnormality is the arrhythmia which makes the rest of the ECG quite difficult to interpret. There are a few sinus beats with a normal PR interval. The normally conducted QRS complexes are rather low voltage and have a normal frontal QRS axis. There are some ST segment and T wave abnormalities in I. The rhythm is almost certainly a ventricular tachycardia; it is broad complex with no prior P wave and is uniphasic in most leads.

(b) An oesophageal lead will enable the P waves to be seen more easily and thus their relationship to the QRS complexes. An alternative procedure would be to place a pacing catheter in the right atrium in order to obtain the same information. Special care is required when performing these procedures in order to ensure that the ECG machine you are using is isolated electrically from the patient; leakage current could have serious untoward effects.

(c) The choice of first line drugs would include an orally active class 1 drug or a class 2 drug such as a beta-blocker. Class 3 drugs such as amiodarone should be reserved as a second line should the other choices not work.

27 (a) The midline scar of the sternotomy and pronounced gynaecomastia.

(b) Spironolactone and digoxin.

(c) The breasts can become painful.

28 (a) She has an extra digit on her left hand together with some hypoplasia of the fifth finger.

(b) Polydactyly can be associated with congenital heart disease.

(c) Yes. The two best known conditions in which polydactyly occurs in association with congenital heart disease are Laurence-Moon-Biedl syndrome and Ellis-van Creveld syndrome. The former is inherited as a recessive and is associated with obesity, mental retardation, renal problems and retinitis pigmentosa. The latter is inherited as a recessive.

29 (a) The xanthelasma are composed of lipid.

(b) She has an obvious arcus. In a young woman the presence of an arcus is highly suggestive of an underlying lipoprotein abnormality.

(c) On the basis that she has been shown to have significant hypercholesterolaemia it is important to do the following: (i) check that she does not have any other risk factors for coronary artery disease, if she does then these need treatment or advice; (ii) embark on the appropriate treatment for her lipid abnormality, in the first instance this will be dietary but she will almost certainly need to have drug treatment as well; (iii) her first degree relatives must also be checked for lipid abnormalities and any other risk factors.

30 (a) Le main d'accoucheur is produced by inducing latent tetany by occluding the arterial supply to the forearm (Trousseau's sign).

(b) The QT interval will be prolonged; this interval will need to be corrected for heart rate (QTc).

(c) Ventricular arrhythmias occur; one of the described arrhythmias is the 'torsade de pointes' which may be mistaken for a conventional ventricular tachyarrhythmia; it is important to recognize it since its treatment differs markedly from that of the conventional ventricular tachyarrhythmia.

31 (a) There is considerable widening of the mediastinum; the appearances are more in keeping with enlargement of mediastinal glands rather than a vascular cause. The heart is also a little enlarged but the lung fields are clear.

(b) She has the classic signs of tamponade: a paradoxical pulse, an inspiratory rise in the venous pressure and a tachycardia. Treatment by pericardiocentesis is urgently required to relieve the tamponade.

(c) With the given story and investigations a lymphoma is the most likely aetiology. Tuberculosis must not be overlooked as a possibility.

(d) The paradox is that as the patient inspires, the heart rate increases but the pulse rate apparently reduces or disappears.

32 (a) He has one of the mucopolysaccharidoses. He has type II (McKusick's classification) or Hunter's disease; this is inherited on a sex-linked recessive basis.

(b) Hepatosplenomegaly, dorsolumbar kyphosis, progressive joint stiffness, swelling and contractures.

(c) There is deposition of the glycoprotein in both the myocardium and in the valves, particularly the mitral valve.

33 (a) They are xanthelasma.

(b) Xanthelasma in this age group are often not associated with any lipid abnormality nor with any vascular disease.

(c) An arcus at this age is of no significance. The prevalence of an arcus rises with age; in women over the age of 50 an arcus is just as likely to be associated with normal or low levels of lipids as with high. There is no association with vascular disease.

34 (a) The ECG shows sinus rhythm with a normal PR interval. The mean QRS axis is markedly to the left. There are deep pathological Q waves in II, III, aVF, V1-4.

(b) The patient has sustained damage to the inferior and anterolateral surfaces of the heart. It is likely that he has disease of both his right and anterior descending coronary arteries; alternatively if the posterior descending was a branch of his circumflex, then he could have disease in the two branches of the left coronary artery. Conclusions about LV function will rest upon the history, physical examination and perhaps exercise testing.

(c) The most important task is to try to determine the age of the infarct. If it was recent, the risks of surgery are significantly increased; if it were possible the operation should be deferred for six months. If one is assured that the infarct is old then it is wise to recommend that the rhythm of the patient is monitored during the operation and that undue hypotension is avoided.

35 (a) The ECG shows sinus rhythm with a normal PR interval. The mean QRS axis is towards the right and is +110 degrees. There is poor R wave progression across the chest leads. There is an extremely short QT and QTc interval with virtual obliteration of any ST segment. There is also generalized flattening of the T waves. The ECG is consistent with hypercalcaemia; the QRS axis raises the possibility of some RV hypertrophy.

(b) The chest condition could be a carcinoma or, more likely, sarcoid giving rise to hypercalcaemia. If there were extensive lung involvement then RV hypertrophy might be expected to develop.

36 (a) She has tendon xanthoma.
(b) Severe hypercholesterolaemia can present with an arthropathy which will affect the ankle joints particularly but can also involve other joints. Xanthoma are usually present in the achilles tendon.
(c) She has the heterozygous form of familial hypercholesterolaemia (FH). She therefore has only half the number of effective LDL receptors on her cell membrane. As a result, the intracellular level of cholesterol is low thus stimulating the further production of cholesterol; these factors produce the high blood levels and the tissue deposition.

37, 38 (a) Meningococcal septicaemia. This condition can be rapidly fatal. It would be useful to know whether there were any other cases of meningococcal infections around. Having taken throat swabs and blood for culture, clotting screen, white count and for the antigen, intravenous antibiotic treatment should be immediately started. The drug of choice is intravenous penicillin in a dose of 4 mega units six hourly.
(b) The low blood pressure is an ominous sign. It is related to the endotoxaemia. Although the occasional case may develop adrenal haemorrhage and the Waterhouse-Friderichsen syndrome, the vast majority have a normal adrenal response to stress. The meningococcus endotoxin is a most potent endotoxin in producing damage to cutaneous blood vessels. The measures to control the hypotension include expansion of the plasma volume and inotropes. The central venous and left atrial pressures may need to be kept quite high since impaired cardiac function may be a consequence of the endotoxaemia.
(c) It is important to trace contacts of the patient and to treat them or vaccinate them as appropriate.

39 (a) Sinus rhythm with a normal PR interval; normal QRS axis widespread upwardly concave ST segment elevation without any reciprocal ST segment depression. These changes are very suggestive of pericarditis.
(b) There are quite deep Q waves in III and aVF together with a dominant R wave in V1; this raises the possibility of an inferior infarct. However the Q waves are probably within normal limits and the dominant R wave relates to the rotation of the heart in the horizontal plane.
(c) Although called acute benign pericarditis it can proceed to tamponade and death. This is an unusual complication but nevertheless needs to be watched for.

40 (a) There is a single ventricle. In the view through the atrioventricular valves both the mitral and tricuspid valves are seen but there is no interposed IV septum.
(b) The single ventricle functions as a common mixing chamber for both saturated and desaturated blood.
(c) The condition can be associated with pulmonary stenosis or atresia. It may be associated alternatively with asplenia.

41 (a) The ECG shows a sinus tachycardia with a normal PR interval. There are pathological Q waves with ST segment elevation in the inferior and lateral leads. There is reciprocal ST segment depression in I and aVL.

(b) The cause of the hypotension must first be elucidated. Extensive myocardial necrosis is only one of the possibilities. An important one to diagnose is that of a low left ventricular filling pressure; this may be caused by the venodilatation caused by opiates or the diuresis that may have been caused by strong diuretics such as frusemide. Both these last two problems will respond to a fluid challenge; the high venous pressure must not put one off this line of therapy, it is probably caused by the infarct involving the right ventricle. If the hypotension is on the basis of a large infarct then treatment will be determined according to the measurement of the left atrial filling pressure and may involve the use of inotropes or vasodilators or both.

(c) It is now thought that the reciprocal ST segment depression reflects a large infarct. At one stage it was thought that it might represent coronary artery disease in another territory; this has now been largely disproved.

42 (a) The ECG shows a sinus tachycardia with a normal PR interval. There is a S1, Q3, T3 pattern. The QRST complexes are otherwise normal. This ECG is normal for someone who is pregnant. There is no evidence of acute right heart strain.

(b) There is a 30 per cent increase in the circulating volume and cardiac output; this starts early in pregnancy and reaches a plateau at the end of the first trimester. It remains elevated for the remainder of the pregnancy and does not decrease in the last trimester as was once thought. There is also a reduction in the systemic resistance resulting in a lowered blood pressure.

(c) The circulating blood volume and cardiac output increase by a further 30 per cent; this begins to fall over the first few hours but, particularly if the mother is breast-feeding, does not return to the pre-pregnancy levels for some weeks.

43 (a) The ECG shows sinus rhythm with a normal PR interval. The QRS axis is about +110°; there is evidence of marked RV hypertrophy with dominant R wave in V1 and V4R together with S waves in the left precordial leads.

(b) The absence of cyanosis and marked RV hypertrophy makes pulmonary stenosis without a septal defect the most likely diagnosis. A reversed shunt is not likely in the absence of cyanosis.

(c) A pulmonary valvotomy or valve replacement is required soon. The symptom of fainting on exertion is a symptom associated with severe stenosis.

44 (a) A very dilated aortic root. There is a clearly seen flap extending from just above the aortic valve around the arch and down the descending aorta. This is the interface between the true and the false lumens. He has a dissection starting in the classical site just above the aortic valve and extending down the descending aorta and also up the carotid artery. This is a type I dissection.

(b) The first measures are to stabilize the blood pressure and ensure the systolic is in the region of 100 mmHg; in this man hypertension was not a problem. Beta-blockers are also used in order to reduce the shearing force of systole. After delineating the type of dissection and the site of the tear, the treatment of choice in this instance is surgical.

(c) Systemic hypertension, Marfan's syndrome and pregnancy.

45 (a) A normal sized heart. The ascending aortic shadow looks fairly normal but the arch and the descending aorta look abnormal; this is the so-called reverse 3 sign of a coarctation. She also has rib notching which is best seen in the 6th-10th ribs posteriorly.

(b) The hypertension is in the upper part of the body only; she had a delayed femoral pulsation and a blood pressure in her legs of 105/85/85 mmHg. The systolic murmur was arising from her bicuspid aortic valve. She also had a systolic murmur that was later in its timing and was maximal between the scapulae; this arises from the blood flow through the coarctation.

(c) Bicuspid aortic valve; congenital berry aneurysm of brain arteries; heart muscle disease.

46 (a) The end-diastolic pressure in the left ventricle is elevated; the left atrial pressure is elevated; there is a large V wave or systolic wave in the LA tracing.

(b) The elevated end-diastolic pressure is indicative of heart failure. The large systolic wave, which is much larger than the A wave, reflects mitral regurgitation. It is difficult, with the limited history and other information given, to be certain of the diagnosis. The patient had a dilated cardiomyopathy and then developed quite severe mitral regurgitation. The patient subsequently had a successful mitral valve replacement and his symptoms improved considerably.

(c) A ruptured chordae; the patient also had a mitral valve that had myxomatous degeneration. Other causes to consider are infective endocarditis, papillary muscle dysfunction and a dilated valve ring associated with the cardiomyopathy.

47 (a) The ECG shows a regular tachycardia which is probably a sinus tachycardia. There are marked ST segment elevation in I, II, III, aVF with ST segment depression in V2. The QRS axis is normal for this age and there is no evidence of any chamber hypertrophy.

(b) A myocarditis is the most likely explanation. An anomalous coronary artery origin from the pulmonary trunk is worth considering but does not usually present in this manner. The child was confirmed to have a Coxsackie B myocarditis.

(c) Heart failure in this age group can be caused by a myocarditis which may be due to the Coxsackie virus or echovirus. Other causes include congenital heart disease; aortic regurgitation; congenital complete heart block or supraventricular tachycardia may also cause heart failure as may arteriovenous shunts. Endocardial fibroelastosis usually presents a little later but can present at this early age. The majority of infants who develop heart failure within the first week of life will do so as a result of critical obstruction of systemic arterial flow such as aortic atresia or coarctation.

48 (a) Aortic valve stenosis; supravalve aortic stenosis; subvalve aortic stenosis; coarctation of the aorta. An obstructive cardiomyopathy would produce a pressure difference between the LV cavity and the outflow tract but the femoral pulse tracing would be expected to be more 'jerky' in character than the one displayed.

(b) The pressure difference is about 75 mmHg which is severe.

(c) Lower. The normal aorta relaxes to accommodate the expressed volume of blood from the ventricle during systole. During systole the aorta recoils thus helping the propulsion of blood distally; this results in the apparent paradox of the femoral artery pressure actually being slightly higher than the aortic pressure.

49 (a) On the PA film the right hilum is abnormal. There is a smooth rounded mass at the right hilum which appears to have blood vessels joining it. There may be similar but smaller lesions at the left hilum. On a lateral the rounded mass can be seen at the hilum; again vessels appear to be joining it. The heart is slightly enlarged. The most likely explanation is that these lesions are vascular and are pulmonary arteriovenous fistulae.

(b) Cardiac catheterization and angiography. A pulmonary angiogram would display the lesion.

(c) The manifestations and complications depend on the size and number of the AV malformations. If large they can present in infancy with cyanosis and heart failure. They can be multiple and part of the Rendu-Osler-Weber syndrome. The other complications are those associated with cyanosis.

50 (a) This is an atrial myxoma. It usually arises and is attached to the interatrial septum. As it grows so it develops a stalk. It can interfere with the function of the mitral valve. It can, as in this woman, be responsible for cerebral emboli.

(b) It can mimic mitral valve disease. It can produce intermittent obstruction of the mitral or other valves. It can sometimes present as a low grade fever and mimic infective endocarditis. It can present as an embolic problem.

(c) 2-D echocardiography is the best investigation. Angiography is now rarely required.

51 (a) Aortic valve.

(b) The valve is likely to have caused obstruction to outflow as well as remaining as a relatively fixed orifice which could not close in diastole. The murmurs were mid-systolic of a crescendo–decrescendo type and an immediate diastolic.

(c) The valve is calcified and this was apparent over the vertebrae on the PA film. The ascending aorta was prominent reflecting the post-stenotic dilatation. The heart was not enlarged since stenosis was the dominant lesion and hypertrophy does not usually produce enlargement of the cardiac silhouette.

52 (a) The aortic valve, shown in the view on the left, is producing a lot of echoes. This is consistent with a thickened or calcified aortic valve.

(b) The pattern of movement of her mitral valve suggests an elevated end-diastolic pressure; the typical M-shaped movement of the anterior leaflet and the W-shaped movement of the posterior leaflet is deformed by a slurring of the final apposition of the leaflets. In the view on the right the walls of the left ventricle are not ideally demonstrated; the wall movements do not appear to be very vigorous and suggest that ventricular function is impaired.

(c) Doppler techniques in conjunction with echocardiography can give information about flow as well as about structure. Some estimate of the actual gradient across the valve can be made with this technique. Systolic time intervals can be used to help make an estimate of the gradient and can be useful if there is difficulty in distinguishing if it is the LV function rather than the aortic valve problem that is predominant. Other non-invasive means must also embrace the physical examination, the ECG and the chest X-ray.

53 (a) Nodal, or more accurately junctional bradycardia. Normal QRS axis. Evidence of inferior myocardial infarction which could be recent. T wave changes over the anterior leads.

(b) Atropine 0.3mg intravenously and repeated if appropriate up to a total dose of 1.2 mg. This usually is sufficient to block the vagal tone and allow a faster heart rate to develop with an improvement in perfusion.

54 (a) Sinoatrial node branch; right ventricular branch (also called acute marginal); branch to AV node; posterior LV branch; posterior descending branch.
(b) The right coronary artery has some disease in it; the walls are a little irregular but there are no critical stenoses. There is cross-filling to the anterior descending territory; this is consistent with disease in this artery. Unfortunately the collaterals do not prevent angina but may reduce the likelihood of a large myocardial infarct in that territory.
(c) The mortality rate will vary with the population under study. If a high proportion of patients studied have mild disease or normal arteries then the mortality will be very low. In Britain the mortality is about 2 in 1000 studies.

55 (a) There are a number of different rhythms recorded. In the top strip the rhythm is complete AV block with a very slow ventricular rate. The following strip shows some coupled ventricular premature beats. The next few strips show a ventricular tachyarrhythmia; this is mostly a ventricular fibrillation. The pattern of the ventricular fibrillation is that of a 'torsade de pointes'. The vector of the QRS complexes changes progressively. It is important to recognize this arrhythmia as its treatment varies from that of a conventional fibrillation.
(b) In the absence of a contraindication she should be treated by permanent pacing.
(c) Asystole is usually the initial rhythm abnormality in patients with complete AV block. Ventricular fibrillation can be a secondary phenomenon but is not usually the initiating rhythm abnormality.

56 (a) Towards the apex of the right ventricle. The ventricle is markedly trabeculated and the electrode tip can be found a secure site. The electrode is inserted under fluoroscopic control.
(b) Once the immediate post-insertion period is over there is a need for the pacemaker to be checked at intervals. The patient needs to avoid fiddling with the palpable part of the electrode under the skin. They need to be advised to avoid strong electric fields such as occur at airport check-ins or old infrared ovens.
(c) The threshold is the minimum power required to stimulate the heart. A reasonable threshold will be less than 0.3 to 1.0 volts with a current of 0.3-2.0 mA at the time of insertion. The threshold usually rises a little after insertion but should not continue to rise. The most commonly used power source now is the lithium iodine cell which lasts 7-10 years.

57 (a) Enlarged heart; enlarged left atrium; enlarged right atrium; calcification in left atrial wall.
(b) The right atrial border is very prominent; this suggests the presence of tricuspid incompetence. The tricuspid incompetence could be on the basis of rheumatic involvement of the tricuspid valve or it could be secondary to right heart failure due to high pulmonary artery pressures.
(c) The Starr Edwards valve will produce an opening sound; the timing of this will be similar to that of the opening snap of mitral stenosis. The closing sound will occur with the first heart sound.

58 (a) The most important difference is the upper mediastinum which has enlarged. The shape of the enlargement suggests a glandular basis.
(b) An enlarged left atrium can press on the oesophagus and cause dysphagia.
(c) Histology is important to obtain. It is unlikely that either bronchoscopy or endoscopy will give this. A mediastinoscopy and biopsy is probably the most fruitful investigation.

59 (a) The X-ray shows a large heart. The pulmonary arteries are all large which suggests a left to right shunt.
(b) It was a continuous murmur of a patent ductus arteriosus. It was well heard in the pulmonary area but was also loud under the left clavicle.
(c) The definitive investigation would be cardiac catheter study and angiography. The study would show a step up in oxygen saturation at pulmonary artery level. The size of the left to right shunt can be calculated. In this instance there was a pulmonary/systemic flow ratio of 4:1. The aortogram demonstrated the duct in the classic site.

60 (a) It is difficult to comment on the heart size in a PA erect film. There is soft intra-alveolar shadowing in both lung fields. This is very suggestive of pulmonary oedema. A pneumonic process is an alternative but the bilateral nature and the hilar flare are against this.
(b) On the basis that this is pulmonary oedema the next question is to determine whether it is related to heart failure or to other causes. The gallop rhythm and haemodynamic changes suggest that it is due to heart failure. An acute myocarditis is a possibility and the recent chest infection would be consistent with this; the ECG is against this diagnosis. A prolonged arrhythmia must be excluded as must a metabolic problem causing the acidosis. A recent myocardial infarction can be easily excluded as a cause. Acute mitral regurgitation might cause a picture of severe pulmonary oedema; however there was no murmur.
(c) It is most unusual not to get some response to the described measures. The severe degree of acidosis and resistant heart failure must raise the possibility of thiamine deficiency. He had Shoshin beriberi and responded dramatically to thiamine.

61 (a) The heart is enlarged, there is a small aortic knuckle and the pulmonary arteries are all very large proximally. They suddenly reduce in size at their tertiary branching. The findings are consistent with a left to right shunt, a high pulmonary vascular resistance and pulmonary arterial hypertension.
(b) She has a left to right shunt. With the given information an ASD is the most likely; the mid-diastolic murmur results from flow across the tricuspid valve.
(c) She has developed pulmonary hypertension as a result of the large left to right shunt. She has now reversed her shunt. Cardiac surgery to close the lesion would actually shorten her life span. The only surgery that could now be considered is that of heart and lung transplantation.

62 (a) Although it is an erect portable film, the heart appears large. The mediastinum is very wide. There is some shadowing at the left base which may be fluid.

(b) A dissection of the aorta is a distinct possibility with his story and the chest X-ray. Previous X-rays would be useful for comparison. His blood pressure needs to be brought down with intravenous nitroprusside infusion to a systolic of 100 mmHg. Beta-adrenoceptor blocking drugs should be given to reduce the shearing stress to the aorta.

(c) The investigation of choice will depend on the local facilities. An echocardiogram might be able to demonstrate the dissection if it involves the aortic root. A CT scan is a very useful investigation. An aortogram should only be done in a cardiothoracic centre but will give the necessary information for the surgeon.

63 (a) The ECG shows Wolff-Parkinson-White syndrome type B. The Q waves in III and aVF are part of this syndrome and do not represent a myocardial infarction.

(b) His dizzy spells may be due to a tachyarrhythmia which is likely to be a reciprocating atrial tachycardia.

(c) Digoxin should be avoided since it enhances conduction down the accessory bundle.

64 (a) The waves are: (i) the a wave related to atrial contraction; (ii) the x descent related to atrial relaxation and the downward movement of the AV valves; (iii) the v wave related to atrial filling; (iv) the y descent related to ventricular filling; (v) the c wave related to the downward movement of the AV valves; (vi) the h wave related to a high diastolic pressure.

(b) There is a strikingly sharp y descent.

(c) Constrictive pericarditis. An alternative might be a tricuspid incompetence but one would expect a large systolic wave preceding the y descent.

65 (a) She has a normal sized heart. The shape of the left heart border suggests an enlarged left atrium and pulmonary artery. There is upper lobe diversion indicative of a raised left atrial pressure.

(b) She has mitral stenosis and a high left atrial pressure.

(c) Atrial fibrillation; systemic embolization; pulmonary arterial hypertension; haemoptysis; pulmonary oedema.

66 (a) The interventricular septum is very thick. The anterior leaflet of the mitral valve is fluttering.

(b) The fluttering of the anterior leaflet is caused by aortic regurgitation. He has the murmur of aortic regurgitation and an Austin Flint murmur.

(c) The regurgitant jet of blood through the leaking aortic valve impinges on the open anterior leaflet of the mitral valve causing it to flutter in a characteristic way.

67 (a) Although this looks like ventricular fibrillation it is often resistant to the therapy that you would normally use. It is a 'torsade de pointes'. The serum potassium must be checked and corrected if necessary. DC version may have a temporary effect. Drugs that prolong the QT interval should be avoided since they tend to make matters worse.

(b) It is worth trying the effect of treating the patient with a drug such as isoprenaline given intravenously. Overdrive pacing is another way of handling this problem; the pacemaker rate is set well above the inherent rhythm and it effectively suppresses the ectopic focus.

(c) Complete AV block. Drugs that prolong the QT interval such as quinidine, procainamide, amiodarone, phenothiazines, and insecticides. Hypokalaemia or hypomagnesaemia. Congenital QT prolongation.

68 (a) A systolic murmur in the phonocardiogram. In the echocardiogram there is a thick IV septum, systolic anterior movement (SAM) of the mitral valve and early closure of the aortic valve. There is also a reduced diastolic closure rate of the mitral valve.
(b) Hypertrophic obstructive cardiomyopathy.
(c) Treatment is necessary to try to reduce the progress of the hypertrophy and also to prevent arrhythmias. The former may be helped by calcium channel blocking drugs, the latter by drugs such as amiodarone or beta-blockers. If the patient has angina then the beta-blocker drug is of particular value.

69, 70 (a) Infective endocarditis. There are numerous vegetations on the mitral valve.
(b) 30 per cent of patients with this condition still die. If the initial presentation is with a neurological picture such as a 'stroke' or confusional state, the risk of death is in excess of 50 per cent. In the elderly the risk of death is about 50 per cent. The longer the interval between the onset of symptoms and the diagnosis and initiation of good treatment, the worse the outcome.
(c) First consider the possibility of infective endocarditis, then examine the patient carefully for clinical evidence of the condition. The next step is to take two or three sets of blood cultures; the ideal time to take these is on the rise of the temperature. There is little to be gained in taking more than three cultures. Examination of a specimen of fresh urine for red cells is also a useful investigation. Although an echocardiogram can confirm a diagnosis, a negative test does not exclude the possibility.
(d) Intravenous antibiotics. The particular antibiotic will depend on the clinical picture and the bacteriological evidence. The adequacy of treatment must be checked with the aid of the microbiologists and the use of back titration techniques. These test whether serial dilutions of the patient's serum will inhibit and kill the actual organism isolated. The duration and route of administration of the antibiotics will depend on this information.

71 (a) The ventricle is large and poorly moving. The mitral valve is only opening with atrial systole. The aortic root is not moving which is consistent with a poor cardiac output. The aortic valve leaflets float together during systole; this also suggests a poor output.
(b) The patient has a dilated heart with very poor LV function.
(c) A postviral cardiomyopathy or alcohol excess are possibilities. Even in the absence of angina or other evidence of coronary artery disease, this picture could be caused by coronary artery disease. In most patients the specific aetiology cannot be determined.

72 (a) The echo shows a large left atrium and a normal sized aortic root. The aortic valve appears normal. The LV dimensions are normal and the wall movements are normal. The mitral valve is abnormal; it is thickened and has a slow diastolic closure rate. The posterior leaflet moves anteriorly with the anterior leaflet in diastole; this is due to commissural fusion. This echo shows mitral valve stenosis.

(b) Yes. Because of the high left atrial pressure the patient is more prone to chest infections and they will tend to last longer than normal. There is interference with lymphatic drainage and this may also play a part.

(c) No. The echo gives anatomical information only. It does not give accurate information about the severity of mitral stenosis.

73 (a) A very loud first heart sound; a close opening snap; P2 is loud, a long diastolic murmur with presystolic accentuation.

(b) The very close opening snap (0.06 sec) and the long murmur suggest that this is severe mitral stenosis. The loud P2 suggests that there is pulmonary hypertension.

(c) The cardiac output and circulating blood volume start to rise soon after the beginning of pregnancy and reach the peak by the end of the tenth week. They then remain constant and do not reduce. At the time of delivery the cardiac output increases by another 30 per cent. The danger times for a lady with mitral stenosis is therefore near the beginning of pregnancy or very soon after delivery.

74 (a) An early systolic click; an early diastolic click; a short systolic murmur after the systolic click.

(b) The clicks are produced by prosthetic valves such as a Starr–Edwards valve. The aortic prosthetic valve will produce the systolic click and short systolic murmur. The mitral prosthetic valve will produce the diastolic click as the valve opens.

(c) These prosthetic valves may produce emboli and the patient has to be anticoagulated. They may produce haemolysis. Very occasionally the ball or the tilting mechanism may get stuck in a particular position. They are of course prone to get infected but no more so than a diseased valve, a homograft or a heterograft replacement.

75 (a) High right ventricular pressure; slightly high right atrial pressure; step up in oxygen saturation at ventricular level; step down in oxygen saturation at left ventricular level; desaturated blood in aorta.

(b) Pulmonary stenosis and a ventricular septal defect; the Fallot situation.

(c) Polycythaemia; gout; high viscosity; endocarditis; paradoxical emboli; syncope; arrhythmias may lead to death.

76 (a) Slow rising pulse with a small notch on the upstroke; soft first sound; soft second sound; systolic murmur.

(b) Aortic valve stenosis.

(c) With the use of systolic time intervals. There are several measurements that can be made; these include the pulse upstroke time, the time to reach half the full upstroke, the pre-ejection period and the ejection time. These measurements will give some indication of the severity of the valve obstruction and also about LV function.

77 (a) Aortic valve is thickened; left atrium is large; mitral valve is thickened and has reduced diastolic closure rate; IV septum and LV posterior wall are thickened.

(b) Aortic stenosis and mitral valve disease.

(c) The aortic valve disease may be severe in the light of the amount of LV hypertrophy. The mitral valve disease is difficult to assess; the large left atrium may be due to the rheumatic process rather than to severe regurgitation. The mitral stenosis is likely to be mild since the posterior leaflet is moving in the normal direction.

78 (a) Elevated LVEDP (diastolic pressure); elevated PA wedge pressure; elevated pulmonary artery and right ventricular pressures.
(b) A myocardial problem.
(c) Idiopathic cardiomyopathy; alcoholic heart disease; coronary artery disease; postviral; drug-related, eg cobalt or duanorubicin.

79, 80 (a) There is coagulation necrosis present. This is characterized by the presence of the dead fibres which are hyaline and structureless. This appearance develops after about eight hours of the event. Subsequent changes include the invasion by polymorphs, and after a few days the digestion by macrophages. The dead muscle is then replaced by fibrous tissue.
(b) Occlusion of a coronary artery causing myocardial infarction.
(c) The coagulation necrosis is evident at about eight hours. There are a number of histochemical markers that have been used to try to determine much earlier changes. Although not entirely reliable, the use of nitroblue tetrazolium or triphenyl tetrazolium chloride can detect ischaemic myocardium at three hours after the event.

81 (a) Pulmonary plethora and a slightly enlarged heart.
(b) The PDA puts a volume load in the left ventricle. Only when pulmonary vascular disease develops does the right ventricle have an additional load.
(c) Surgical management. The heart is already large because of the volume load and needs to be relieved of it.

82 (a) With the given story the most likely sequence is that of fat emboli leading to hypoxia; the analgesia made this worse causing a hypoxic cardiac arrest. The other possibility might be related to the withdrawal effects from alcohol; a chest infection in these circumstances is not unusual and could produce hypoxia leading to the arrest. Although there is no suggestion of a head injury, it obviously must be excluded.
(b) After fat emboli the two most difficult complications to deal with will be disseminated intravascular coagulation or the adult respiratory distress syndrome. The withdrawal effects from alcohol or other drugs can be very difficult to manage in a sick patient.

83, 84 (a) An isotope that passes through the capillary network and is accumulated intracellularly is required if the presence of ischaemia is to be determined. Thallium is the commonly used isotope for this purpose. It has the ability to substitute biologically for ionic potassium thereby accumulating rapidly within viable cells. It has a low energy spectrum and a half-life of 73 hours.
(b) There is poor perfusion of the anteroseptal part of the left ventricle which reperfuses slightly at rest; this represents his old infarct together with some reversible ischaemia.

85 (a) There is a large mass within the left atrium which moves down towards the left ventricle on the lower frame. It is almost certainly a left atrial myxoma. It could be a different form of tumour. The valve looks quite normal.
(b) Embolic phenomena are very common. The diagnosis should be at least considered in every patient presenting with an embolism.
(c) Surgical removal.
(d) The tumour may recur. There may also be other members of the family with a myxoma.

86 (a) The patient is in atrial fibrillation. There is an echogenic mass moving through the mitral valve in diastole and back into the left atrium in systole. The valve cusps themselves look normal and are not thickened. This could be an atrial myxoma or other cardiac tumour.

(b) Mitral regurgitation can occur because of the interference with the mitral valve function by the tumour. The movement of the tumour can produce an audible 'plop' which can be confused with an opening snap.

(c) The narrow single beam makes the interpretation of anatomy difficult. It takes a well trained technician to produce good and reliable results. There is a need to learn to recognize the pattern of the tracing in contradistinction to 2-D where the actual movements of structures are visualized.

87 (a) It shows sinus rhythm with a normal PR interval. The P wave is tall particularly in II, III, and aVF. There is marked right axis deviation. There is a dominant R wave in V1 and S waves in V5-6. These changes suggest right atrial and right ventricular hypertrophy.

(b) Syncope.

88 (a) There is sinus rhythm with a short PR interval and a delta wave. He could be misdiagnosed as having an infarction.

(b) Although he has the Wolff-Parkinson-White syndrome a diagnosis of myocardial infarction will need to be excluded by other means such as enzymes. He actually had dyspepsia.

89 (a) Sinus rhythm with a normal PR interval. Changes of an acute inferior myocardial infarction with reciprocal changes in the anteroseptal leads.

(b) They reflect a large infarct. They do not appear to reflect coexisting disease in that territory as was once thought.

(c) In an inferior infarct he may have a high right atrial pressure because of infarction of the right ventricle; his left atrial pressure may be low. He may therefore respond to a fluid challenge.

90 (a) The ECG is normal. Although there is quite a lot of voltage (R in V6 + S in V1 > 35 mm); this is normal for a slim, healthy young man.

(b) A normal ECG does not rule out the possibility of a cardiovascular problem. The test is very non-specific and care has to be taken in either ascribing too much or too little importance to it.

91 (a) The high sampling rates from the two piezoelectric crystals makes the continuous wave doppler an ideal technique for recording high flow velocities.

(b) Pulsed doppler. In this mode there is only one piezoelectric crystal which alternates as a transmitter and a receiver. A burst of ultrasound is emitted by the transducer which then receives the signals from the depth of interest. The return signal is analysed for doppler shifts for a very brief time period; accordingly shifts in frequency can be determined very accurately at specific points along the beam. Its limitation is its relatively slow sampling rates for high velocity flow.

(c) Yes. The flow is towards the transducer and therefore shown above the line. Normal flow through an aortic valve may be 1.0-1.5 m/sec. In this instance the maximum flow is less than this; the aortic stenosis can be presumed to be minimal. Poor LV function may reduce the flow through a diseased aortic valve and therefore cause its severity to be underestimated.

92 (a) The waveform in systole is laminar and reflects flow through the aortic valve. There is also diastolic spectral broadening characteristic of aortic regurgitation.

(b) The aortic systolic flow is approximately 2 m/sec which is slightly increased and suggests the presence of mild aortic stenosis. Quantification of regurgitant lesions is more difficult; in regurgitation there is a jet of blood flowing from a high pressure area into a low pressure. As a result there is a high velocity laminar jet of flow in the regurgitant orifice itself together with a flow disturbance in the chamber receiving the flow. To try to judge the severity a technique termed flow mapping is used. This requires pulsed doppler and the sample volume probe is sited and sampled in different regions of the appropriate chamber. This enables a picture to be built up of the spatial relationships of the regurgitant flow. If the flow disturbance is only present in the plane below the valve, then mild regurgitant is present; if the flow disturbance is distributed widely then severe regurgitant is present. The size of the chamber into which the jet flows will also have an influence on the flow characteristics.

(c) The introduction of colour flow doppler enables more accurate estimation of the characteristics of flow. It is still at a relatively early stage of technological development.

93 (a) Atrial flutter with 4:1 AV conduction.

(b) It produces characteristic flutter waves in the venous pulse in the neck.

(c) Because of varying AV block the ventricular rate changes suddenly; the patient finds this rapid change very difficult symptomatically.

(d) The choice is between synchronized DC shock and drug therapy. If DC shock is used it will usually need very small energy levels; sometimes only 20 joules are needed. Digoxin will reduce AV conduction and protect the ventricles from very fast rates; it may convert the rhythm to atrial fibrillation which the patient may find more satisfactory.

94 (a) Sinus rhythm with atrial premature beats.

(b) The treatment of her pain and distress is likely to reduce the likelihood of ventricular fibrillation. The serum potassium should be checked and corrected if necessary. There is no good evidence that drug therapy actually reduces the likelihood; in this lady any anti-arrhythmic drug is likely to reduce her blood pressure further and may actually increase the likelihood of VF.

(c) She has a very extensive infarct; the most likely reason is that she has little remaining LV myocardium. However it is important not to miss treating an inappropriately low filling pressure of her left ventricle; remember that the injured LV will require a higher filling pressure than normal.

95 (a) He has the Wolff-Parkinson-White syndrome. It is possible that prolonged arrhythmias may have contributed to his heart failure. He has not had an inferior infarct.

(b) The only drug that one would avoid using is digoxin because of its adverse influence on the development of the reciprocating arrhythmias. Otherwise the treatment choices involve the vasodilators, an ACE inhibitor, diuretics, xamoterol or a phosphodiesterase inhibitor.

96 (a) It is difficult to be 100 per cent certain with this sort of rhythm. However there are a number of features which suggest that it is ventricular in origin: monophasic V1; mean QRS axis towards the left; wide bizarre complexes.

(b) DC shock is a very effective treatment. One of the difficulties with drug treatment is that most of the effective drugs for a ventricular arrhythmia are negative inotropes. If they successfully convert someone back to a normal rhythm then the negative inotropic effects are not important; however if the drug does not work, the patient may become more ill.

(c) After trying the various tricks at the bedside such as carotid sinus massage, Valsalva's manoeuvre, and different electrode positions there are two techniques that are worth trying. An underused technique is that of an oesophageal lead; it enables the atrial activity to be readily seen and its relationship to ventricular activity identified. An alternative is to use a pacemaker electrode and place the tip in the right atrium in order to record atrial activity.

97 (a) Loud first heart sound; systolic murmur; opening snap.

(b) She has mitral valve disease.

(c) The accurate timing of clicks and snaps. In most other ways the well trained human ear is superior.

98 (a) The left atrium is very large. The enlargement may be because of the raised pressure in the left atrium; it is perhaps more likely to be as a result of left atrial myocardial involvement by rheumatic fever.

(b) The mitral valve. The reduced amplitude of excursion, the reduced diastolic closure rate and the anterior movement of the posterior leaflet are due to the fibrosis, thickening, tethering and commissural fusion that occur as a result of the rheumatic process.

(c) Yes. The interventricular septum does not move normally. This is because of the splinting effect of the rigid mitral valve.

99 (a) The left atrium is large; there is splaying of the carinal angle, there is the bulge on the left heart border and there is a double density shadow to the right of the vertebral column. It is much more difficult to be certain about other chamber enlargement. The right atrium may be enlarged but it could just be pushed across by the left atrium. One of the ventricles is likely to be enlarged; on the basis that the clinical details are known, it is possible to deduce which one. Without the clinical details one cannot tell on the PA film and there is difficulty even with the help of a lateral.

(b) Upper lobe blood diversion gives information of the left atrial pressure; if it is present the left atrial pressure is likely to be at least 18 mmHg. Septal lines also indicate an elevated left atrial pressure.

100 (a) She has a marked scoliosis. This makes the interpretation of the heart shape and size difficult. However she does have a large heart. There is also quite a marked difference in the upper and lower lobe veins. The large heart suggests either a volume load on the ventricle or a myocardial problem. The upper lobe blood diversion suggests a raised left atrial pressure.

(b) This combination would fit for mitral regurgitation or a left ventricular myocardial problem.

101 (a) On the PA film the heart shadow may appear large.
(b) A systolic murmur may be found together with delayed closure of the pulmonary valve.
(c) Right bundle branch may be found.

102 (a) A large heart. There is also a fat pad which makes the heart appear even bigger. There is no evidence of a raised left atrial pressure.
(b) On the information given, it seems likely that he has an infection or perhaps a malignant process. The combination of a high venous pressure in someone who is comfortable lying flat raises the possibility of pericardial constriction.
(c) An echocardiogram will confirm the presence of pericardial fluid; it will not help determine the haemodynamic consequences of this fluid. A lateral X-ray of the chest can indirectly contribute to the diagnosis of pericardial fluid by inspection of the fat pad. Appropriate investigations will need to be performed to diagnose tuberculosis; pericardial aspiration is unfortunately often unhelpful in this regard.

103 (a) Bilateral flare from the hila. This is very suggestive of acute left ventricular failure.
(b) A rapid onset of shortness of breath suggests a number of possibilities; however most of them would assume some prior underlying problem which was apparently absent in this man. A silent, acute infarct could present in this way but he is rather young for this. A ruptured chordae could account for this picture; pre-existing mitral valve disease would be likely. If there had been a story of chest trauma, an acute valve problem could have resulted. An arrhythmia superimposed on impaired left ventricular function would be a possibility if he had not been previously fit. An acute myocarditis is unlikely to present so dramatically. A myocardial toxin might cause such a presentation; cobalt used to make beers more frothy can present this acutely. Other toxins include scorpion venom, poisoning with phosphorus or arsenic, and drugs such as adriamycin. The heart may be affected in anaphylaxis induced by drug sensitivity and can present in this way.
(c) The patient should respond to standard treatment for heart failure unless there is some irreversible process such as described above.
(d) A condition that must not be overlooked since it is so easily treated is thiamine deficiency. It can present acutely like this and may be made worse if you are keeping a vein open with a dextrose infusion.

104 (a) Aortic regurgitation. She has a large heart suggesting a volume load on the ventricles; the shape of the enlargement is consistent with aortic regurgitation. The ascending aorta is quite prominent suggesting an aortic valve problem. One cannot rule out a coexisting mitral regurgitation; the left atrium is not enlarged however.
(b) This can be extremely difficult to determine with aortic regurgitation; the volume load is well tolerated by the heart and surgery should not be performed too early. The ideal time for surgery is just before there is evidence that the heart is beginning to suffer. You should be looking for evidence of an enlarging ventricle; serial echocardiographic examination is probably better than X-ray. Evidence of ECG deterioration is useful although not so good a guide as in aortic stenosis. The patient's symptoms should not be the determining factor; they tend to be late and the ideal timing is past.

105 (a) Left coronary artery.
(b) The left main stem divides into: anterior descending, circumflex. The branches of the anterior descending include septal branches, diagonal branch(es). The branches of the circumflex include the marginal branches posterior left ventricular branches and, in some patients, the posterior descending branch and the branch to the AV node.
(c) Yes. The anterior descending supplies the proximal bundle branches and the bundle of His. In 20 per cent of people the circumflex gives rise to the AV nodal branch.
(d) Yes. The anterior two-thirds is supplied by the anterior descending; in the 20 per cent whose circumflex gives rise to the posterior descending, the posterior third of the septum will be supplied by this branch.

106 (a) A very large heart. There is no evidence of a raised left atrial pressure.
(b) A pericardial effusion. The aetiology is difficult to predict without more clinical information.
(c) Sometimes the pericardial effusion can cause tamponade. This needs to be treated as a medical emergency with aspiration of fluid.

107 (a) The mitral valve has been replaced.
(b) A mitral xenograft or homograft valve.
(c) The xenograft (different animal species) and homograft (same animal species) valves are more physiological and do not require anticoagulation. In a woman who may want to get pregnant the problems associated with anticoagulation are best avoided if possible.

108 (a) The aortic valve. The fact that it is difficult to see in the PA film means that it is overlying the vertebral column. If it were in any other valve position it would be to the side of the vertebral column and therefore more easily seen.
(b) Some models of the S E valve last for ever and outlive the patient. In most patients this valve will last in excess of 15 years.
(c) The mortality is about 1 per cent per annum. The morbidity is considerably higher. It is also an inconvenience for the patient and adversely affects the quality of life.

109 (a) Sinus rhythm; normal PR interval and QRS axis; left ventricular hypertrophy; ST segment and T wave abnormalities; these are non-specific.
(b) The P wave in V1 is predominantly negative; this implies a raised left atrial pressure. It is quite a sensitive index. It will become less negative as the patient improves with treatment.

110 (a) There is marked ST segment depression of >2 mm in the anterior and inferior leads. He has generated a heart rate of 145/min.
(b) It is likely that he will be shown to have significant disease in three vessels.
(c) We need to know the haemodynamic response; did his blood pressure continue to rise or not? This will give information about left ventricular function. We need to know whether he got chest discomfort. There is a lot of potential information in an exercise test which can be lost or ignored if the test is merely reported as being positive or negative.

(d) The risk is very small; the mortality rate is about 1 in 20,000 and infarction rate 1 in 3000. It is therefore important that patients are appropriately screened before a test and that resuscitation equipment and a doctor is available nearby.

111 (a) On the stress images there is hypoperfusion of the inferior surface of the heart. There is some reperfusion at rest but this is not complete. It is likely that there is some reversible ischaemia in the inferior part of the heart but there is also some old myocardial necrosis in this territory.
(b) The posterior descending coronary artery.
(c) In the inferior leads.

112 (a) It is very abnormal. Only a very small part of the ventricle has a good amplitude of movement.
(b) No. There is a large segment of the left ventricle which is not in phase.
(c) This is very low.
(d) The ejection fraction of the contracting segment (CS EF) is shown to be 32 per cent. This raises the possibility that, by removing the LV aneurysm, the remaining left ventricle may cope better; indeed it may improve the overall function of the ventricle and improve the symptoms of the patient.

113 (a) Sinus rhythm with a normal PR interval. Right bundle branch block.
(b) Very difficult to tell in the presence of right bundle branch block. Vector cardiography might be able to differentiate.
(c) Her pulmonary sound is likely to be soft and delayed; the second sound will therefore be widely split but moving appropriately.

114, 115 (a) The PA chest X-rays show a massively dilated and tortuous descending thoracic aorta. The sternal wires from the previous operation are present. The heart size itself is large.
(b) The major anxiety in this type of major operation is that of a paraplegia; even in the best hands the risk of this is in the order of 5-8 per cent and the mortality rate is about 15 per cent.
(c) Control of any systemic hypertension is vital. The use of a beta-adrenergic blocking drug is also valuable in order to reduce the shearing force on the vessel wall.
(d) Atherosclerosis is the most likely to affect the aorta in this way. Others to be considered would be: (i) syphilis: this usually affects the ascending aorta; (ii) cystic medial necrosis: this also usually affects the ascending aorta; (iii) a dissection: this can affect the descending aorta and spare the ascending aorta; it may be associated with (ii).

116 (a) The diastolic pressures in the two ventricles are raised and are very similar, the two atrial pressures are similar and both are raised, the right ventricular and pulmonary artery systolic pressures are raised.
(b) The similar filling pressures of the two ventricles is very suggestive of constrictive pericarditis. If there were a left ventricular problem only, the LV diastolic pressure would be elevated more than the RV which might be normal. A restrictive cardiomyopathy might produce this pattern but again one would expect some differentiation in the pressures between the right and left side of the heart.
(c) She had a constrictive pericarditis; surgical removal is the treatment of choice.

(d) The constriction of the pericardium affects both ventricles and atria; the haemodynamics are thus very different to those which pertain with left ventricular disease. In the latter, the very different right and left ventricular function curves cause the symptom of orthopnoea.

117 (a) There is a very severe pressure difference between the right ventricle and the pulmonary artery. This pulmonary stenosis may be at valve level or at subvalve or both.
(b) She will have an abnormal JVP with a dominant 'a' wave. The JVP may not be elevated. There will be RV hypertrophy manifest by a parasternal heave. There will be a systolic murmur maximal in the pulmonary area which will not radiate to the neck; it will not be a pansystolic murmur; it may be associated with a thrill. If the obstruction is at valve level there may be an ejection click. The second heart sound will be abnormal; P2 may be delayed or absent.
(c) She probably had a paradoxical embolism.
(d) On exertion her right atrial pressure will exceed her left atrial; right to left shunting then takes place through an ASD or patent foramen orale.

118 (a) This is a Dotter basket catheter.
(b) It has been introduced in order to snare and then remove the remains of a central venous catheter which has floated into the right ventricle.

119 (a) This is a normal ECG.
(b) If there is no historical lead, or an abnormality on examination, routine ECGs are unhelpful. Indeed they can be positively dangerous in that they induce a false sense of security. The argument that they are useful in hindsight should something happen is weak, and does not help with the acute management of any presenting problem.

120 (a) The mitral valve ring is thickened; the anterior leaflet of the mitral valve has a reasonable excursion but a very slow diastolic closure rate (E-F slope) and is thickened; the posterior leaflet is not well demonstrated but moves posteriorly during ventilation systole.
(b) The loud first sound is shown and is coincident with mitral valve closure; a quite late opening snap corresponds to the opening of the mitral valve; the lateness of the opening snap and the relatively normal movement of the posterior leaflet are consistent with relatively mild stenosis. The M-mode must not be relied upon as an index of severity.
(c) The patient is in atrial fibrillation. The most likely cause is an embolus.
(d) Anticoagulants will prevent further embolic episodes; however there is a risk of introducing them too soon after a cerebral event. If there is evidence of structural damage as manifest by a neurological deficit lasting longer than 24 hours, the initiation of anticoagulants should be delayed; there is debate about the delay but some will argue that it should be at least six weeks. The risk of causing a bleed into the ischaemic or infarcted area exceeds the risk of a further embolus. If there is a full recovery after the transient episode, that early introduction of oral anticoagulants is indicated. If the clinical assessment is of mild mitral stenosis, then there is no indication for surgery which is usually determined on haemodynamic grounds.

121 (a) Large left ventricular cavity; poor movement of LV walls; small pericardial effusion; late opening of mitral valve; poor movement of aortic root; cusps of aortic valve float together during systole; slightly large left atrium.

(b) This appearance could be caused by a congestive cardiomyopathy; the pathology would be very non-specific. It might be secondary to a myocarditis; if there was still an active inflammatory process than there might be an inflammatory cell infiltrate together with the fibrotic scarring. It might be caused by coronary artery disease.
(c) The heart murmur will be due to mitral or tricuspid regurgitation secondary to the dilatation of the left or right ventricles.

122 (a) The ECG shows a normal pacemaker artefact and normal pacing from the right ventricle,
(b) Yes. He will have reversed splitting of his second heart sound; he effectively has a left bundle branch block.

123 (a) The ECG is highly suggestive of an acute inferior myocardial infarct. There is slight but definite ST segment elevation in the inferior leads with some ST segment depression in aVL.
(b) We need a little more information before knowing how best to proceed. Although a myocardial infarct remains the most likely diagnosis she could have a major pulmonary embolus. Sometimes an acute abdomen may present in this way and have these ECG changes. If the latter two conditions can be excluded with a fair degree of certainty, then the decision must be made about the use of aspirin together with streptokinase, anistreplase or tPA in the context of someone who has peptic symptoms. If there had not been recent symptoms and no bleeding then enteric coated aspirin and the thrombolytic drug can be given. The evidence of benefit with an inferior infarct is not as dramatic as with an anterior; nevertheless there is still some benefit.

124 (a) Atrial flutter, varying AV block. right bundle branch block, Q waves in inferior leads.
(b) On the basis of the ECG the possibilities might be: (i) the inferior infarct may be quite recent and caused the faint; (ii) the onset of atrial flutter or a change in AV conduction may have caused a temporary reduction in cerebral perfusion.
(c) If shown to have a recent infarct then he will need the appropriate treatment; in this age group extremely early mobilization is wise. In the absence of a proven infarct, it is important to try to document whether a recurrent arrhythmia is the mechanism of the faint by 24 hour ambulatory recordings.

125 (a) Sinus rhythm with evidence of an anterior myocardial infarct; the timing of the latter is difficult but it could have occurred two weeks ago.
(b) The operation should be postponed. The risk of surgery after a recent myocardial infarction is high; this risk remains for some six weeks and the operation should, if possible, be deferred until after this period has elapsed.

126 (a) The ECG is normal apart from a right bundle branch block. The complexes are all of rather small voltage.
(b) A RBBB can be a normal finding; the low voltage may be on the basis of her overweight. If you think that her heart is normal then she can continue to hold the PSV licence. If there is any doubt in your mind, then further investigations need to be performed to clarify the situation.

127 (a) Wide splitting of the second heart sound; early systolic murmur; a RBBB on the ECG. There is some AC interference on the ECG. The baseline is not very satisfatory in diastole; the appearance just before the first heart sound is caused by tricuspid closure and there is no diastolic murmur.

(b) An atrial septal defect. It is difficult with the amount of information given to be certain that the second heart sound is relatively fixed in its splitting. The second component of the split sound is not an opening snap; you can identify the aortic closure because it occurs just before the dichrotic notch on the pulse tracing; the sound after the notch must therefore be pulmonary closure.

(c) If the shunt through the ASD were large, a tricuspid flow murmur would be expected.

128 (a) The right ventricle may be large. The movement of the interventricular septum may move in an abnormal and paradoxical fashion; this allows the large RV volume to be accommodated. In the four chamber view the interatrial septum may be visualized; if the ASD is large then the defect may be visualized. If saline or dextrose is injected into a peripheral vein the micro-bubbles will be visualized as they pass through the right atrium and the the right ventricle; they do not appear on the left side normally since they are 'filtered' by the lungs. In an ASD there will be some right to left shunting and the micro-bubbles will be seen to pass from RA to LA.

(b) It is a superior investigation because: (i) better anatomical information is obtained; (ii) it is an easier technique to learn and to obtain reliable information; (iii) in conjunction with doppler studies it will give both the anatomical information and also information about blood flow and velocity of flow; the echo is used to direct the doppler beam to the point of interest.

(c) The value of the 2-D image is best appreciated on video tape recordings where the moving image is recorded. Still frames for reproduction lose a lot of their quality; this does not apply for the M-mode.

129 (a) Sinus rhythm with a normal PR interval. The QRS axis is posteriorly orientated. There is a dominant R wave in V1 and S waves in V5 and V6. These changes suggest right ventricular hypertrophy.

(b) There is no mention of any cyanosis and therefore a right to left shunt is unlikely; to present with syncope suggests the presence of pulmonary vascular disease and therefore some right to left shunting. Nevertheless knowledge of the size of the proximal pulmonary arteries would be of value. Radiological evidence of lung disease or evidence of pulmonary emboli should be sought. Even though there is no diastolic murmur, evidence of a raised left atrial pressure should be sought.

(c) Was she taking the oral contraceptive pill? Had she been taking any slimming remedies?

(d) The pulmonary artery pressure could be measured; the absence of any shunt can be confirmed and the left atrial pressure shown to be normal. The pulmonary vascular resistance can then be calculated.

130 (a) Raised pulmonary artery pressure; raised right ventricular systolic and diastolic pressures; large 'a' wave in RA trace.

(b) Primary pulmonary hypertension. Thromboembolic pulmonary hypertension. Pulmonary hypertension due to high altitude or lung disease is unlikely due to the extreme level of the pulmonary artery pressure.

c) High concentrations of oxygen are only of temporary value. Certain vasodilators such as nifedipine or the angiotensin-converting-enzyme inhibitors may have a role which is occasionally dramatic. If a precipitating factor can be identified then it should be removed. Heart and lung transplantation is available for those patients who do not respond to these measures and who are suitable in other ways.

31 (a) Acute anterior myocardial infarction.
b) Yes. Intravenous streptokinase, anistreplase (APSAC) or tPA given promptly may cause the ECG to revert to normality.

32 (a) The picture shows an occluding thrombus in a coronary artery.
b) It is now recognized that in a large proportion of patients, the formation of an intraluminal thrombus plays an important part in a myocardial infarction. The rupture of the fibrous cap covering the atheromatous plaque allows the passage of blood into the intima with the formation of a thrombus and resulting in expansion of the plaque. There also is the development of thrombus within the lumen; this does not necessarily occlude the lumen but initially waxes and wanes in size. If the thrombus occludes the vessel for long enough a myocardial infarction ensues.
c) Yes. The use of both aspirin and a fibrinolytic drug are of proven benefit so long as they are used within a few hours of the occlusion.

33 (a) Loud pulmonary valve closure. Soft first heart sound. Systolic murmur occupying the whole of systole and with a crescendo–decrescendo character. Sharp upstroke to arterial pulse.
b) The mitral valve. The murmur is shown to start with the soft first sound and to spill over into early diastole through the second heart sound.
c) Mitral valve prolapse with severe mitral regurgitation. It is unlikely to be a rheumatic aetiology because of the absence of a diastolic murmur.
d) She probably ruptured a chordae causing more severe mitral regurgitation; this is a well described complication of this condition.

34 (a) The fluttering is found in aortic regurgitation; this is caused by the regurgitant jet impinging on the open mitral valve in ventricular diastole. It can also sometimes be found in mitral regurgitation.
b) The left ventricular cavity is very large. The LV walls move poorly. There is no hypertrophy of the LV walls.
c) His poor left ventricular function is associated with a raised end-diastolic pressure producing shortness of breath.
d) If his main problem had been valvular incompetence, regular follow up is intended to identify the point in time when his left ventricle begins to fail; ideally to identify when it is about to start failing. However in this instance the lack of LV hypertrophy suggests that it is actually the LV dysfunction, rather than valvular incompetence that is the main problem. If there had been any evidence of ongoing activity of the rheumatic process then treatment should have been instituted.

35 (a) Paget's disease of bone.
b) If a considerable proportion of the skeleton is involved, an increased cardiac output and increased pulse pressure may occur. This is related to the multiple, small arteriovenous fistulae. A heart murmur due to the increased flow may therefore occur.
c) Atrioventricular block may sometimes be associated with this condition as can cor pulmonale.

136 (a) High end-diastolic pressure in left ventricle. Marked variation in systolic pressure in the presence of a sinus tachycardia.
(b) He has acute tamponade with a paradoxical pulse. It is likely that he sustained an aortic dissection.
(c) The pericardium is attached to the great vessels well above the aortic valve. The intimal tear in the aorta can enable blood to track down in the false lumen to below this pericardial attachment and blood will thus enter the pericardial space.

137 (a) Low pulmonary artery pressure; high infundibular pressure; very high pressure in the body of the right ventricle; pressure difference or gradient at valvular and infundibular levels.
(b) The patient probably has Fallot's tetralogy and the cyanosis is on the basis of right to left shunting at ventricular level.
(c) Squatting. This raises systemic resistance and enhances pulmonary flow thereby.
(d) Surgery. Both the valvular and infundibular obstructions can be relieved and the VSD closed. The patient will still have residual abnormalities in the right ventricular outflow tract and will continue to need to be followed in a medical clinic. The patient should continue to take precautions for any septic procedures.

138 (a) Yes.
(b) Yes. The aorta overrides the interventricular septum; this is best seen in the top left tracing. Normally the anterior wall of the aorta is continuous with the septum. In this patient the septum appears to end in the centre of the aorta; this is the overriding aorta.
(c) Tetralogy of Fallot.

139 (a) In the left ventricle.
(b) The catheter has passed from IVC→→RA→→LA→→LV. The passage through the interatrial septum is either through a patent foramen ovale or through an ASD.
(c) About 30 per cent of normal people have a patent foramen ovale; in theory therefore this passage of the catheter can occur.

140 (a) Papilloedema; multiple flame shaped haemorrhages; numerous exudates.
(b) Systemic hypertension. Because of the changes in the optic fundi this used to be called malignant hypertension; perhaps now better labelled accelerated hypertension.
(c) Prior to the introduction of effective hypotensive agents, all patients presenting with hypertension and these fundoscopic changes were dead within five years; if they had haemorrhages and exudates without papilloedema the five year survival was only 13 per cent.
(d) Since the advent of effective hypotensive agents the prognosis is considerably better. The outlook for patients will depend on the aetiology of the hypertension, the extent of target organ damage already existing and the ease with which good blood pressure control can be achieved.

141 (a) Sinus tachycardia on the top strip, ventricular bigemini on the second strip, one couplet of ventricular beats on the third strip.

(b) The histogram summates the heart rate over a defined period. It is particularly useful when information concerning the heart rate over the 24 hour period is needed, for instance in a patient with atrial fibrillation. If a patient has an ectopic focus producing a tachycardia, the histogram gives information about the proportion of the day that the ectopic focus dominates the heart rate. In this patient there is a normal histogram which embraces the day time and night time heart rates. The histogram on the left is bimodal; the mode on the left represents the short RR interval when the patient has ventricular bigemini.

142 (a) Very high chylomicron levels. The patient has a rare deficiency of lipoprotein lipase which is inherited on an autosomal recessive basis. The triglyceride levels are also elevated.
(b) Because the serum is clear, one can assume that the triglyceride levels are normal. The serum cholesterol is elevated.
(c) Since the serum is opalescent one can assume the triglyceride levels are elevated. No deduction can be made about the cholesterol level which may be high, low or normal.

143 (a) He has a normal sized heart. The arch of the aorta is abnormal; the shape is characteristic of someone with a coarctation showing the reversed 3 sign. There is well shown rib notching.
(b) There may be an associated bicuspid aortic valve. Congenital berry aneurysms are also thought to be associated.
(c) In this condition there is often a typical marked tortuosity of the arterioles.
(d) The blood pressure may rise steeply.

144 (a) A large bulge on the left heart border which represents an LV aneurysm.
(b) Heart failure; arrhythmias; emboli; rupture.
(c) Echocardiogram; ideally two-dimensional. Radioisotope studies. Angiography, fluoroscopy, clinical examination.

145 (a) Long PR interval (1st degree AV block), voltage criteria of left ventricular hypertrophy.
(b) The combination of aortic regurgitation and a long PR interval is suggestive of an aortitis such as ankylosing spondylitis or Reiter's syndrome.
(c) In these conditions the inflammatory process and adventitial thickening spreads down from the aorta to involve the membranous ventricular septum and the base of the mitral valve. It can therefore involve the conducting system.
(d) Manifestations of the arthropathy, eye changes etc.
(e) A high proportion of individuals afflicted have the HLA-B27 antigen.

146 (a) SAM; systolic anterior movement of mitral valve during systole. Very thick and immobile interventricular septum.
(b) Hypertrophic cardiomyopathy with obstruction.
(c) Syncope usually occurs after exertion in contradistinction to aortic valve stenosis in which it occurs during the exertion.
(d) An autosomal form of inheritance has been described. It is therefore important to screen the first degree relatives.

147 (a) The echocardiogram is normal. You need to see the video in order to give a proper report.

(b) There is no evidence of endocarditis. However the echocardiogram cannot rule out the possibility of the diagnosis which has to be made on other criteria.

148 (a) Atrial fibrillation with a very fast ventricular response. QRS axis of about +5 degrees. Generally rather low voltage QRS complexes with poor R wave progression across the precordium. Widespread non-specific ST segment and T wave abnormalities.
(b) Her ventricular rate needs to be controlled and her left ventricular function improved. After checking her serum potassium, digoxin will be a useful drug but its dosage will need careful control. Diuretics in a lady of this age need to be used with care because of the urinary problems that they will cause her. A mild vasodilator might be a more suitable drug for her.

149 (a) Sinus bradycardia; J waves; long QT interval.
(b) Hypothermia.
(c) Reduced intake whilst becoming hypothermic; polyuria due to tubular dysfunction in hypothermia; rewarming producing vasodilatation.

150 (a) Technetium (99^mTc labelled albumen) is usually used for the perfusion scan. Xenon gas (^{133}Xe) is used for the ventilation scan.
(b) The intention of the investigation is to determine whether there are any areas of the lung that are ventilated and not perfused; this will be suggestive of pulmonary emboli, the probability being in the order of 90 per cent. Areas that are neither perfused nor ventilated may occur in atelectasis, asthma, pneumonias or vasculitides.
(c) There are perfusion defects seen in both lungs which are not matched by ventilation defects; the left lung perfusion defects are seen in all three views. The right lung perfusion defect is seen in the posterior view.
(d) In the ventilation scan the trachea is usually outlined.

151 (a) Suspicion of an aortic dissection.
(b) The intimal flap is well seen both in the ascending aorta and the descending; it gives the latter the appearance of a tennis ball. The flap can also just be seen in the arch of the aorta.
(c) The origin of the dissection should be identified; this is of great help in the further management. If the origin of the dissection can be confidently diagnosed, this may obviate the need for an aortogram.
(d) The dissection may well have involved a coronary artery; this may cause spasm or actual blockage.
(e) After the pain has been relieved and the blood pressure adequately controlled, the next stage in the management is to identify the type of dissection. If the tear originates in the ascending aorta, the next step is surgical. If the tear is distal to the origin of the left subclavian, the care is medical in the first instance.

152 (a) The ascending aorta and the descending aorta have an intimal flap demonstrated; this results from a dissection of the aorta.
(b) The left atrium.
(c) Pulmonary veins.
(d) The descending aorta.

153 (a) An enlarged heart. The lung fields look normal.
(b) He may have underlying heart muscle disease.

(c) He may be HIV positive; he will thus be predisposed to infections which may make endocarditis more likely. There is also some evidence that, in the absence of infections, heart muscle disease occurs in these patients; this may be on an immunological basis.

154 (a) A large heart; large proximal pulmonary arteries; no peripheral 'pruning' of pulmonary vessels.
(b) A left to right shunt. The level is difficult to determine without more information. The most likely shunt at this age would be an ASD.
(c) There is a large shunt as manifest by the size of the pulmonary vessels. Surgical correction of the shunt is the preferred treatment.
(d) If there were to be a high pulmonary vascular resistance then surgery would be contraindicated. This seems unlikely in this case because of the lack of pruning.

155 (a) There is some confluent shadowing in the right middle and lower zones of the lung.
(b) The tip of the nasogastric tube is seen in the right lower lobe bronchus; the enteral feeding has entered the lung causing the radiographic changes and her symptoms.
(c) Removal of the nasogastric tube and energetic physiotherapy.

156 (a) Enlarged heart; large left atrium; some shadowing at the left base.
(b) The left atrium which is extremely large.
(c) Rheumatic heart disease.
(d) A heterograft or xenograft; this is tissue from another animal species. The usual one used is a pig. A homograft or valve from the same animal species. An autograft or valve from the same person; the valve from another site can be switched. A prosthetic or man-made valve; there are a variety of designs and makes of these.

157, 158 (a) There is an enlarged left atrium. The heart size is normal. There is upper lobe blood diversion.
(b) The left atrium is enlarged. There is no valve calcification.
(c) With an enlarged left atrium there is a risk that certain medication may be held up in the oesophagus and cause local damage; this particularly applies to Slow K tablets. The only other gut problem is, of course, embolic to the gut arteries.
(d) The temptation immediately to anticoagulate the patient must be resisted. The risk of anticoagulation and thus causing bleeding into the ischaemic brain is high and is present whether the initial event was thrombotic, embolic or a haemorrhage. Although somewhat controversial the author recommends that the interval between the event and the initiation of anticoagulation should be at least four weeks.

159 (a) A large heart; a large left atrium; upper lobe blood diversion. Some shadowing at both his bases.
(b) It is likely that he has mitral regurgitation. In the absence of any history to suggest endocarditis, the most likely problem is that of degeneration of his mitral valve causing chordal rupture and the development of severe mitral regurgitation.
(c) Echo/doppler studies will give structural information about the mitral valve together with information about ventricular size and wall movement. The doppler will give information about the severity of the mitral regurgitation.

(d) Mitral valve surgery; valve replacement is probably preferable unless the surgeon is very experienced and skilled at valve repair.

160 (a) First degree heart block; partial right bundle branch block; left axis deviation with left anterior hemi-block.
(b) Development of complete AV block with associated episodes of asystole or ventricular fibrillation.
(c) Insertion of permanent pacemaker.

161 (a) The rhythm is sinus rhythm with atrial premature beats followed by a compensatory pause. The chest leads are artefactual.
(b) The chest leads are missing; the standard leads have been mounted twice instead.

162 (a) The ECG is recorded at the wrong paper speed; in this instance it is recorded at 10 mm/sec instead of 25 mm/sec. There are abnormal T waves in V6. There is also voltage criteria of left ventricular hypertrophy.
(b) Repeat the ECG at a normal paper speed.

163 (a) This is a MUltiple Gated Acquisition (MUGA) scan.
(b) The principle of the scan is to use the R wave of the ECG as the triggering signal. The radionuclide data from the injected radioisotope is collected and segregated temporarily into 16 to 28 equal divisions or pixels, depending on the heart rate. Studies require from 2 to 10 minutes for completion. A left and right ventricular time-activity curve is based on analysis of the left anterior oblique position. To obtain information about regional wall movement, several different views are required.
(c) Atrial fibrillation or frequent and persistent ectopic activity makes the study virtually impossible. The inability of the patient to lie still also makes the study difficult.
(d) There are several circumstances in which this investigation can give useful information. In the patient being considered for surgery, an accurate estimate of their ejection fraction will aid the decision-making process. In the patient with an aneurysm, this study will give a good estimate of the function of the remaining LV.
(e) This scan shows generally very poor ventricular function. The amplitude image shows poor amplitude of left ventricular wall motion. The phase image is extremely fragmented demonstrating discoordinate ventricular contraction. The ejection fraction of each ventricle is in the order of 6–8 per cent. If an operation were being contemplated, the chances of getting him off the operating table would be very low.

164 (a) The aortic valve is heavily calcified; it is difficult to actually see any orifice at all. In this view, one is looking into the aortic valve from above and normally would see it open widely in systole.
(b) The long axis view shows the thickened, calcified aortic valve, and a normal sized LV cavity; the definition of the still frame is not good enough to determine the degree of hypertrophy of the LV walls; the left atrium is enlarged.
(c) She has severe aortic valve stenosis.

(d) The ECG may give some additional indirect evidence of the severity. The physical examination is, of course, the best non-invasive means of all. The doppler/echocardiogram is an extremely useful investigation and can give good information about the severity of this valve lesion. The use of systolic time intervals can also give helpful information.

165 (a) By constructing volume curves throughout the cardiac cycle from each pixel of a gated blood pool scan, colour coded images of amplitude of regional wall motion, and phase of wall motion can be generated. In this example the normal phase image shows that both ventricles contract uniformly and in synchrony (coded green); the atria (coded red) are 180 degrees out of phase. The amplitude image shows vigorous LV contraction.
(b) Yes.
(c) It is a normal study.

166 (a) The rhythm is a junctional one.
(b) At the bedside you should be able to see regular cannon waves.
(c) The oesophageal lead enables you to identify the atrial activity if it is hidden within the ventricular complexes on the surface ECG. Having identified the atrial activity it is then possible to determine its relationship to the ventricular complexes. If you know the siting of the tip of the oesophageal lead (distance from the mouth) then you can, from the shape or vectors of the atrial complexes, determine the origin of the rhythm in the atria.

167 (a) An atrial rhythm; atrial and ventricular asystole; sinus rhythm.
(b) This patient has sino-atrial disease and ventricular conducting system disease. In the light of the symptoms a pacemaker is the preferred treatment.
(c) Conducting tissue disease can be part of a chronic fibrotic process of unknown aetiology. Although it is often associated with coronary artery disease, there is little evidence to demonstrate a cause and effect relationship. In certain parts of the world it can be part of a systemic disease such as Chagas' disease.

168 (a) There is a marked inflammatory response with infiltrates of white cells. There is some destruction of muscle fibres and some early fibrotic changes.
(b) The picture is one of a myocarditis; the most likely aetiology is viral. The commonest viral agents are a Coxsackie B or echovirus.
(c) A myocarditis is a very common complication of any systemic viral illness such as influenza; the vast majority of people recover without sequelae. A small number will go on to develop heart failure and a small group will present with sudden death.
(d) It is very important that energetic exercise is avoided during the weeks following the infection. All too often it is a premature return to strenuous activity that precipitates a demise.

169 (a) MUGA is an achronym for MUltiple Gated Acquisition scan. The technique involves acquiring information over hundreds of cardiac cycles using the R wave as the reference point for the computer acquisition. The RR interval is divided into 16 to 28 equal subdivisions depending on the heart rate.
(b) The isotope has to be reasonably stable; technetium labelled red cells are used.

(c) With the aortic regurgitation, the left ventricular stroke volume is higher than the right ventricular.

(d) Yes. This is one of the virtues of the investigation; an accurate ejection fraction can be obtained. In this instance the left ventricular cavity is enlarged and the ejection fraction is reduced slightly at 55 per cent.

170 (a) His systolic blood pressure should progressively increase with the workload. If his pressure does not increase under this stress, the test should be terminated. A failure of the blood pressure to rise is an indication of a failing ventricle.

(b) We know that he has had an inferior infarct. The ST segment changes in the exercise test suggest significant ischaemia in the anterior descending coronary artery.

(c) An exercise test on a hospital population in Britain will have a specificity of about 85 per cent and a sensitivity of 60 per cent.

(d) The prevalence of the disease in the population under study. This relationship was first described by Bayes who stated that the predictive value of an investigation is variable and depends on the probability of the disease in the population under study. He described this theorem in an essay entitled 'Essay towards solving a problem in the doctrine of chances' in the 18th century.

171 (a) Extremely thick interventricular septum, systolic anterior movement of the mitral valve (SAM), slow diastolic closure rate of the mitral valve, pericardial fluid.

(b) Hypertrophic obstructive cardiomyopathy together with a pericardial effusion.

(c) Typical. Angina is very common in severe forms of this condition. Dizziness or syncope after exercise is also typical and is different from the symptoms that occur with exertion in aortic valve stenosis.

(d) An arrhythmia.

(e) Yes. The condition may be inherited on a dominant basis.

172, 173 (a) Coarctation of the aorta.

(b) The hypertension is much easier to control after the coarctation has been operated upon.

(c) A paraplegia.

(d) Brachial-femoral delay; a late systolic murmur best heard over the scapulae which may spill over into diastole; there may be palpable collateral vessels with an associated bruit.

174 (a) The heart is slightly large. The aortic knuckle is small. The pulmonary arteries to all zones of the lung are large; there is therefore pulmonary plethora. There is no pruning of the pulmonary arteries.

(b) A left to right shunt. We need the clinical information in order to be more precise. The small aortic knuckle is more suggestive of an ASD than the other shunts.

(c) In order to get plethora the shunt has to have at least a pulmonary:systemic flow ratio of 2:1. This is severe enough to cause the development of pulmonary hypertension and reversal of the shunt.

(d) The more precise shunt can be calculated by performing catheter studies and measuring saturations. It is likely that this particular shunt will work out to be at least a 2:1 and more like a 3:1. If the patient had presented at a younger age, surgery would have been advised. She is one of the few patients with a large shunt who go through life without running into serious haemodynamic trouble.

175 (a) The heart is enlarged. The left atrium is large. These appearances suggest mixed mitral valve disease.
(b) The haemoptysis is due to the mitral valve disease.
(c) The circulating blood volume increases by about 30 per cent within the first few weeks of pregnancy and remains at this level until delivery; it then increases by another 30 per cent. The most dangerous time therefore is in the immediate postdelivery period.
(d) A valvotomy can be performed without significant fetal mortality; however if the patient has coped up to three months there is rarely a need and the problems can be managed medically. If bypass is required the fetal mortality rises to 33 per cent. It is best done earlier rather than later if the patient cannot be controlled on medical therapy.

176 (a) A very enlarged heart. The right heart border suggests right atrial enlargement. The film is rather overexposed which makes comments about the vascular pattern in the lungs difficult.
(b) On a PA chest X-ray it is not possible to determine which of the ventricles is enlarged; it may be both. Even with the help of a lateral you will be wrong fairly frequently. Both atria are very large in this patient.
(c) Large atria 'accommodate' severe regurgitation much better than small chambers. As a result the patient remains less symptomatic for longer.

177 (a) Both the limb leads and the precordial leads are suggestive of dextrocardia.
(b) The aortic area and pulmonary areas are transposed; it is actually A2 that is being heard.
(c) Ask the technician to record the ECG again with the arm leads transposed and the precordial leads recorded as V6R, V5R, V4R etc.

178 (a) There is an extremely thick interventricular septum. The posterior LV wall is also thick. The aortic valve looks normal.
(b) Although there is hypertrophy of both the free LV wall and the IV septum, it is likely that the patient has hypertrophic cardiomyopathy which is probably obstructive.

179 (a) The long axis view of the heart.
(b) Thick interventricular septum, echogenic myocardium, pericardial fluid, slightly thickened aortic valve.
(c) There may be an infiltrative process; examples might be amyloid or sarcoid. In this instance the patient had amyloid.

180 (a) A right sided pneumothorax is present. There is shadowing at the right apex, at the right base and hilum. The appearance of these shadows suggest an infective cause; the appearances in the lung suggest that some of the lesions may be cavitating.
(b) The appearances are consistent with embolic infected material causing lung abscesses; they raise the possibility of a right-sided endocarditis with perhaps a staphylococcus as the infecting organism.

(c) Right-sided endocarditis. The clinical diagnosis of a right sided endocarditis is difficult. If the heart had been previously normal, there may be no murmurs. If the tricuspid valve is involved there will be none of the typical signs associated with chronic tricuspid valve disease; there will be no pulsatile liver and perhaps no murmurs. The only abnormal sign may be an abnormal character of the JVP. The diagnosis is made by first considering it. Careful examination of the JVP and careful auscultation may give a lead. Blood cultures are essential. An echocardiogram may demonstrate the vegetations, but their absence does not exclude the diagnosis.

Index

Numbers refer to illustrations

Alcoholic heart disease 78, 82
Amiodarone 26, 68
Amyloid 179
Aneurysm 34, 45, 112, 143, 144
Aneurysmal dilatation 114, 115
Angina 15, 27, 132, 164, 171
Angiography 49, 59
Anistreplase (APSAC) 131
Ankylosing spondylitis 145
Aorta 3, 45, 138, 152; coarctation 16, 25, 48, 172, 173
Aortic dissection 3, 62, 151; regurgitation 104, 114, 115, 134, 145; root 44; stenosis 25, 91; valve 19, 45, 51, 52, 92, 108; *see also* Stenosis
Aortogram 44, 62
Arcus 28, 33
Arrhythmia 7, 15, 26, 75
Arteriogram, coronary 5, 54
Artery 4, 5, 34
Atherosclerosis 114, 115
Atrial fibrillation 7, 65, 86, 96, 120, 148, 157, 158, 163; flutter 93; myxoma 50, 86; pressure 65; septal defect (ASD) 24, 61, 127, 128, 139, 174; tachyrhythmias 11, 30, 63; tachycardia 14
Atrium 98, 99, 152
Austin Flint murmur 66
AV block 2, 9, 56, 67, 135

Beriberi, Shoshin 60
Brachial-femoral delay 172, 173
Bradycardia 53, 166
Bruce protocol 110, 170
Bundle of His 2, 105; block 101, 113, 122, 126, 127
Bypass, saphenous vein graft 1

Cardiac arrest, hypoxic 82; catheterization 24, 49, 75, 78, 129
Cardiomyopathy 46, 121; hypertrophic obstructive 68, 178; idiopathic 78; postviral 71
Cardiovascular system, in pregnancy 42
Catheter, data 75, 78, 81, 116, 117, 130; Dotter basket 118
Cerebrovascular accident 117
Chagas' disease 167
Chest, infection 72, 82; leads 161; pain 53, 136
Chordae, ruptured 46, 103, 133
Chylomicron levels 142
Coagulation, disseminated intravascular 82; necrosis 79, 80

Coronary, arteriogram 5, 54, 105; artery disease 34, 71, 78, 111
Coxsackie virus 47, 168
Cyanosis 13, 137, 138
Cystic medial necrosis 114, 115

DC shock 93, 96
Dextrocardia 177
Digoxin 27, 93, 95, 148
Disseminated intravascular coagulation 82
Doppler techniques 52, 91, 92

Ebstein's anomaly 11
ECG 7, 12, 15, 16, 17, 18, 22, 25, 26, 30, 34, 35, 39, 42, 43, 90, 110, 119, 122, 162
Echocardiogram 20, 23, 66, 120; M-mode 20, 40, 52, 68, 71, 86, 128, 138; 2-D 50, 85, 128
Echovirus 47, 168
Ellis-van Creveld syndrome 28
Emboli, cerebral 13; fat 82; paradoxical 13, 75, 117; pulmonary 18
Endocarditis 75, 147, 180; infective 46, 69, 70
Endotoxaemia 37, 38
Epigastric pain 12, 94, 123
Eye lesions 29, 33

Fallot, tetralogy of 75, 137, 138
Fibrillation, ventricular 55

Gastrectomy, partial 14
Gout 25
Gynaecomastia 27

Haemoptysis 65, 72, 175
Hand abnormalities 30, 36
Heart disease, alcoholic 78, 82, muscle 45, 153, rheumatic 104, 156; and drug addiction 180; failure 13, 60, 109, 121, 148, 156, in neonate 47; large 100, 102; and lung transplantation 61; murmur 11, 12, 19, 23, 25, 28, 32, 43, 46, 48, 50, 51, 52, 59, 65, 66, 68, 72, 73, 76, 77, 87, 100, 117, 121, 134, 135, 146, 154, 156, 178
Heterograft 156
HIV positive 153
Homograft valve 107
Hunter's disease 32
Hypercalcaemia 35
Hypercholesterolaemia 28; familial (FH) 36
Hypertension 62, 160, 172, 173; pulmonary artery 6, 61, 65, 73, 130; systemic 44, 114, 115, 140
Hypertrophy, RV 35, 61, 87, 129
Hyperuricaemia 13
Hypokalaemia 15, 67
Hypomagnesaemia 67
Hypotension 41
Hypothermia 149
Hypovolaemia 15

Ischaemia 111, 152; transient attack (TIA) 120

J waves 15

Laurence-Moon-Biedl syndrome 28
Le main d'accoucheur 30
Lipid abnormalities 142
Lithium iodine cell 56
Lymphoma 31

Marfan's syndrome 44
McKusick's classification 32
Mediastinoscopy 58
Mediastinum 31
Meningococcal septicaemia 37, 38
Mitral regurgitation 100, 134, 139
Mitral stenosis 4, 23, 65, 72, 73, 120
Mitral valve, disease 58, 77, 86, 97; prolapse
    20, 133; prosthetic 57, 69, 70, 98, 107;
    surgery 159; xenograft 107
Mucopolysaccharidoses 32
MUGA (MUltiple Gated Acquisition) scan
    112, 163, 165, 169
Myocardial infarct 10, 22, 54, 79, 80, 83, 84,
    88, 118, 123, 125, 131, 132; inferior 124
Myocarditis 47, 168
Myocardium 79, 80, 179
Myxoma, atrial 50, 85, 86

Nasogastric tube 155
Necrosis, coagulation 79, 80; cystic medial
    114, 115
Neonate, heart failure 47
Nifedipine 130

Oedema 57, 60, 65
OT prolongation 67

Pacemaker 9, 56, 160
Paget's disease of bone 135
Pain, chest 53; epigastric 94, 123
Palpitation 45
Pancreatitis 10, 15
Papillary muscle dysfunction 46
Papilloedema 140
Paradoxical emboli 13, 75, 117
Paradoxical pulse 31
Paraplegia 114, 115
Patent ductus arteriosus 59
Perfusion scan 150
Pericardial effusion 106
Pericardiocentesis 31
Pericarditis, acute benign 39; constrictive 64,
    116
Pneumonia 135
Pneumothorax 180
Polycythaemia 13, 75
Polydactyly 28
Pregnancy 44, 73, 173; cardiovascular system
    in 42
Pulmonary artery pressure 4; emboli 18;
    fibrosis 21; hypertension 6, 61, 65, 73, 130;
    oedema 60, 65; plethora 81; stenosis 40,
    43, 73, 117, 139; vein 24

Radioisotope study 163
Raynaud's phenomenon 21
Reiter's syndrome 145
Rendu-Osler-Weber syndrome 49
Rheumatic fever 63, 66, 77, 91, 98, 134, 176
Rheumatic heart disease 104, 156
Rhythm, gallop 179; sinus 17, 94, 109, 113
RV hypertrophy 35, 61, 87, 129

Scan, MUGA 112, 156, 163; perfusion 150;
    ventilation 150
Scleroderma 21
Scoliosis 100
Septicaemia, meningococcal 37, 38
Shoshin beriberi 60
Shunt, left to right 61, 154, 174
Sino-atrial disease 167
Sinus tachycardia 18, 60, 136, 141
Starr-Edwards valve 57, 74, 108
Stenosis, aortic valve 16, 48, 76, 77, 164;
    mitral valve 23, 65, 72, 73; pulmonary 40,
    43, 117
Sternal depression 101
Sternotomy 27
Streptokinase 131
Syncopal attacks 55
Syncope 75, 87, 146
Syphilis 8, 114, 115
Systolic anterior movement (SAM) 146, 171

Tachyrhythmias, atrial 11, 30, 63
Tachycardia 93; atrial 14; sinus 18, 60, 136,
    141
Technetium 150
Tendon xanthoma 36
Thallium 83, 94
Thiamine deficiency 60, 103
Thrombus 132
Tissue plasminogen activator (tPA) 18, 131
'Torsade de pointes' 30, 55, 67
Transient ischaemic attack (TIA) 120
Transplantation, heart and lung 61
Trousseau's sign 30
Tuberculosis 31, 102

Valsalva's manoeuvre 96
Valvotomy 113, 175
Valvular disease 176
Venous pressure 57
Ventilation scan 150
Ventricular bigemini 141; conducting system
    disease 162; failure 103; fibrillation 55

Waterhouse-Friderichsen syndrome 37, 38
Waves 64; J 15
Wolff-Parkinson-White syndrome 7, 63, 88,
    95

Xanthelasma 28, 33
Xanthomata 10; tendon 36
Xenograft 107, 156
Xenon 150